Resistance to Targeted Anti-Cancer Therapeutics

Volume 17

Series Editor:
Benjamin Bonavida

More information about this series at http://www.springer.com/series/11727

Andrés J. M. Ferreri
Editor

Resistance of Targeted Therapies Excluding Antibodies for Lymphomas

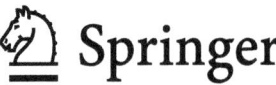
Springer

Editor
Andrés J. M. Ferreri
Department of Onco-Hematology
Unit of Lymphoid Malignancies
IRCCS San Raffaele Scientific Institute
Milan, Italy

ISSN 2196-5501　　　　　　ISSN 2196-551X　(electronic)
Resistance to Targeted Anti-Cancer Therapeutics
ISBN 978-3-319-75183-2　　　ISBN 978-3-319-75184-9　(eBook)
https://doi.org/10.1007/978-3-319-75184-9

Library of Congress Control Number: 2018935142

© Springer International Publishing AG, part of Springer Nature 2018
This work is subject to copyright. All rights are reserved by the Publisher, whether the whole or part of the material is concerned, specifically the rights of translation, reprinting, reuse of illustrations, recitation, broadcasting, reproduction on microfilms or in any other physical way, and transmission or information storage and retrieval, electronic adaptation, computer software, or by similar or dissimilar methodology now known or hereafter developed.
The use of general descriptive names, registered names, trademarks, service marks, etc. in this publication does not imply, even in the absence of a specific statement, that such names are exempt from the relevant protective laws and regulations and therefore free for general use.
The publisher, the authors and the editors are safe to assume that the advice and information in this book are believed to be true and accurate at the date of publication. Neither the publisher nor the authors or the editors give a warranty, express or implied, with respect to the material contained herein or for any errors or omissions that may have been made. The publisher remains neutral with regard to jurisdictional claims in published maps and institutional affiliations.

Printed on acid-free paper

This Springer imprint is published by the registered company Springer International Publishing AG part of Springer Nature.
The registered company address is: Gewerbestrasse 11, 6330 Cham, Switzerland

"Resistance to Targeted Anti-Cancer Therapeutics": Aims and Scope

Published by Springer Inc.

For several decades, treatment of cancer consisted of chemotherapeutic drugs, radiation, and hormonal therapies. Those were not tumor specific and exhibited several toxicities. During the last several years, targeted cancer therapies (molecularly targeted drugs) have been developed and consisting of immunotherapies (cell mediated and antibody) drugs or biologicals that can block the growth and spread of cancer by interfering with surface receptors and with specific dysregulated gene products that control tumor cell growth and progression. These include several FDA-approved drugs/antibodies/inhibitors that interfere with cell growth signaling or tumor blood vessel development, promote the cell death of cancer cells, stimulate the immune system to destroy specific cancer cells and deliver toxic drugs to cancer cells. Targeted cancer therapies are being used alone or in combination with conventional drugs and other targeted therapies.

One of the major problems that arise following treatment with both conventional therapies and targeted cancer therapies is the development of resistance, preexisting in a subset of cancer cells or cancer stem cells and/or induced by the treatments. Tumor cell resistance to targeted therapies remains a major hurdle and, therefore, several strategies are being considered in delineating the underlining molecular mechanisms of resistance and the development of novel drugs to reverse both the innate and acquired resistance to various targeted therapeutic regimens.

The new Series *"Resistance of Targeted Anti-Cancer Therapeutics"* was inaugurated and focuses on the clinical application of targeted cancer therapies (either approved by the FDA or in clinical trials) and the resistance observed by these therapies. Each book will consist of updated reviews on a specific target therapeutic and strategies to overcome resistance at the biochemical, molecular and both genetic and epigenetic levels. This new Series is timely and should be of significant interest to clinicians, scientists, trainees, students, and pharmaceutical companies.

Benjamin Bonavida
David Geffen School of Medicine at UCLA
University of California, Los Angeles
Los Angeles, CA 90025, USA

Series Editor Biography

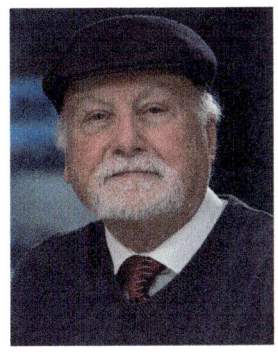

Dr. Benjamin Bonavida, PhD (Series Editor) is currently Distinguished Research Professor at the University of California, Los Angeles (UCLA). His research career, thus far, has focused on basic immunochemistry and cancer immunobiology. His research investigations have ranged from the mechanisms of cell mediated killing, sensitization of resistant tumor cells to chemo−/immunotherapy, characterization of resistant factors in cancer cells, cell-signaling pathways mediated by therapeutic anticancer antibodies, and characterization of a dysregulated NF-κB/Snail/YY1/RKIP/PTEN loop in many cancers that regulates cell survival, proliferation, invasion, metastasis, and resistance. He has also investigated the role of nitric oxide in cancer and its potential antitumor activity. Many of the above studies are centered on the clinical challenging features of cancer patients' failure to respond to both conventional and targeted therapies. The development and activity of various targeting agents, their modes of action, and resistance are highlighted in many refereed publications.

Acknowledgements

The Series Editor acknowledges the various assistants who have diligently worked in both the editing and formatting of the various manuscripts in each volume. They are Leah Moyal, Kevin Li, and Anne Arah Cho.

Editor's Biography

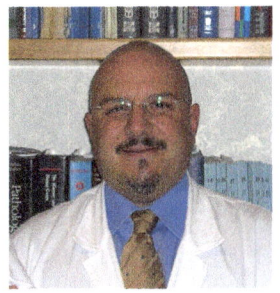

Andrés J. M. Ferreri has a degree in Medicine from the Facultad de Medicina of the Universidad de Buenos Aires, Argentina (1985), and obtained the degree of Doctor in Medicine and Surgery in the Facoltà di Medicina e Chirurgia dell'Università degli Studi di Parma, Italy, in 1992. He is a Specialist in Clinical Oncology (Università degli Studi di Milan, Italy, 2005). He was a research fellow at the Divisione di Oncologia Sperimentale "E" and at the Divisione di Oncologia Médica "A" of the Istituto Nazionale dei Tumori of Milan (1989–1994) and vice-director of the Medical Oncology Unit of the San Raffaele Scientific Institute of Milan, Italy. Currently, Dr. Ferreri is Head of the Unit of Lymphoid Malignancies of the San Raffaele Scientific Institute of Milan, and is a Contract Professor of Oncology in the Vita e Salute University, Milan. He is fully devoted to the research on non-Hodgkin lymphomas and is an opinion leader in the field of extranodal lymphomas. Dr. Ferreri is Associate Editor of the ESO/START Project and of "Haematological Oncology" and Faculty of the European School of Oncology. Dr. Ferreri is a member of EHA, ESMO, ASH, and ASCO.

Preface

Targeted therapies are one of the most important components of the armamentarium against epithelial malignancies. A fast growth of our knowledge of the molecular mechanisms and activated pathways in the different lymphoma categories was followed by a more diffuse and successful use of targeted therapies. Monoclonal antibodies were the first molecules in this field, whereas several other agents targeting different key molecules involved in the activated pathways were investigated and are being used in routine practice. Importantly, most of these agents can be used by the oral route and the assumption for years is not associated with an increased risk of severe side effects. However, long-lasting treatment with these drugs is followed by disease relapse in a high proportion of patients, which is predominantly due to the development of drug resistance. The knowledge of mechanisms involved in lymphoma resistance to target therapies is of paramount importance because it will result in a better selection of patients with sensitive disease, tumor monitoring, relapse prediction, and establishment of combination of drugs that target different molecules that could overcome the established resistance.

This book is focused on recently developed targeted therapies other than monoclonal antibodies used in lymphoma patients, both in routine practice and in investigative trials. Expert authors revisit the most relevant aspects of these agents, with special emphasis on molecular mechanisms and clinical effects of resistance. Although more space is dedicated to the first-in-class members of each drug family, other recently developed agents are discussed.

Milan, Italy   Andrés J. M. Ferreri

Contents

BTK Inhibitors: Focus on Ibrutinib and Similar Agents 1
Mattias Mattsson and Lydia Scarfò

BCL2 Inhibitors: Insights into Resistance 23
Mary Ann Anderson, Andrew W. Roberts, and John F. Seymour

Proteasome Inhibitors with a Focus on Bortezomib 45
Kevin Barley and Samir Parekh

IMiD: Immunomodulatory Drug Lenalidomide (CC-5013; Revlimid) in the Treatment of Lymphoma: Insights into Clinical Use and Molecular Mechanisms 73
Pashtoon Murtaza Kasi and Grzegorsz S. Nowakowski

mTOR Inhibitors, with Special Focus on Temsirolimus and Similar Agents 85
Teresa Calimeri and Andrés J. M. Ferreri

Inhibitors of the JAK/STAT Pathway, with a Focus on Ruxolitinib and Similar Agents 107
Linda M. Scott

Index. 135

BTK Inhibitors: Focus on Ibrutinib and Similar Agents

Mattias Mattsson and Lydia Scarfò

Abstract Since Bruton tyrosine kinase (BTK) is a critical effector molecule for B cell development and lymphomagenesis, BTK inhibitors have been investigated in B cell malignancies during the last decade. Ibrutinib, a first-in-class, potent, orally administered covalently-binding inhibitor of BTK was recently approved for the treatment of chronic lymphocytic leukemia (CLL), mantle cell lymphoma (MCL), Waldenström's macroglobulinemia (WM) and marginal-zone lymphoma (MZL). Its use led to impressive responses in CLL, MCL, WM and MZL with a favorable safety profile. Mechanisms of resistance to ibrutinib are different according to disease biology and still need to be fully elucidated. In CLL and WM patients progressing on ibrutinib, BTK and downstream kinase Phospholipase Cγ2 (PLCγ2) mutations have been identified leading to resistance. BTK and PLCγ2 mutations are almost always absent at the beginning of treatment and they are detected at a later timepoint, suggesting the evolution of clonal dynamics under treatment pressure. Primary and secondary resistances in MCL are driven by mutations promoting the activation of the alternative NFκB-pathway and PI3K-AKT pathway. Further work needs to be done to elucidate the mechanisms behind primary refractory patients, to define the risk for clonal evolution/new mutations over time on treatment, and to identify prognostic/predictive markers for patients on BTK inhibitors.

Keywords BTK inhibitors · Ibrutinib · B cell malignancies · Acalabrutinib · ONO/GS4059 · BGB-3111 · CC-292

M. Mattsson
Department of Hematology, Uppsala University Hospital and Department of Immunology, Genetics and Pathology, Uppsala University Uppsala, Uppsala, Sweden

L. Scarfò (✉)
Università Vita-Salute San Raffaele and IRCCS Istituto Scientifico San Raffaele, Milan, Italy
e-mail: scarfo.lydia@hsr.it

© Springer International Publishing AG, part of Springer Nature 2018
A. J. M. Ferreri (ed.), *Resistance of Targeted Therapies Excluding Antibodies for Lymphomas*, Resistance to Targeted Anti-Cancer Therapeutics 17,
https://doi.org/10.1007/978-3-319-75184-9_1

Introduction

In the last years, several novel findings have strengthened the notion that B cell receptor (BcR) signaling through both antigen-dependent and antigen-independent mechanisms plays a crucial role not only in normal B cell development and survival but also in the pathogenesis of B-cell lymphoproliferative disorders [1].

BCR activation promotes the assembly of the so-called "signalosome" which includes protein tyrosine kinases like Lck/Yes novel tyrosine kinase (LYN), spleen tyrosine kinase (SYK), Bruton tyrosine kinase (BTK), and other kinases, resulting in cell survival and proliferation, differentiation, and antibody production (Fig. 1) [2].

The essential role for BTK in BCR signaling activation is strongly supported by the fact that loss-of-function mutations in BTK block B-cell maturation at the pre-B-cell stage and cause the clinical signs and symptoms of X-linked agammaglobu-

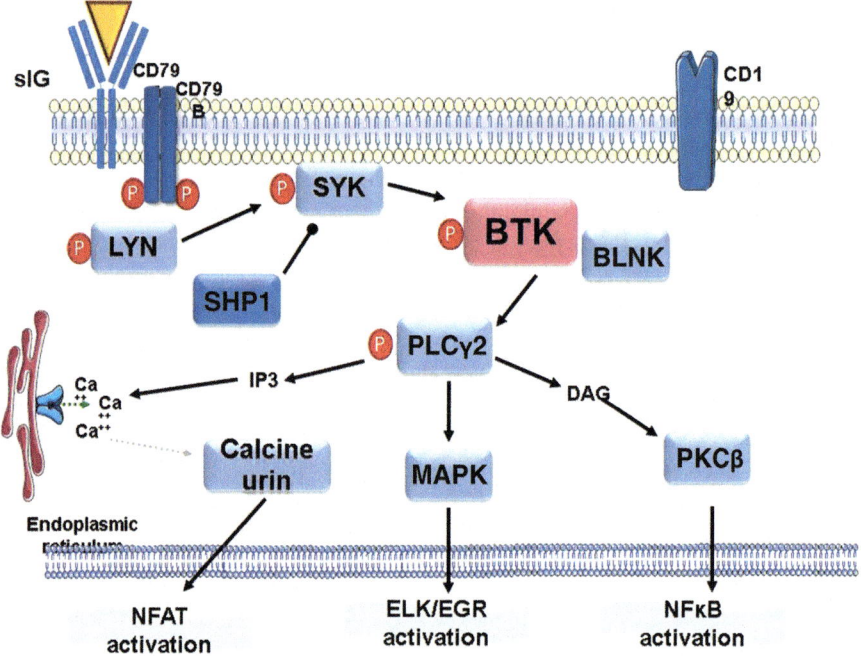

Fig. 1 BTK role after BCR activation. BCR activation promotes the assembly of the so-called "signalosome" which includes protein tyrosine kinases like Lck/Yes novel tyrosine kinase (LYN), spleen tyrosine kinase (SYK), Bruton's tyrosine kinase (BTK), and other kinases mainly represented by phospholipase C-gamma 2 (PLCγ2) and phosphatidylinositol 3-kinase-delta (PI3Kδ). Within the signalosome BTK phosphorylation by LYN and SYK promotes BTK activation. BTK is recruited early in the BCR signaling cascade and upon activation of the BCR pathway. Subsequent PLCγ2 phosphorylation leads to calcium mobilization, ERK, AKT and NFκB activation, resulting in cell survival and proliferation, differentiation, and antibody production. (The figure was produced using Servier Medical Art: www.servier.com)

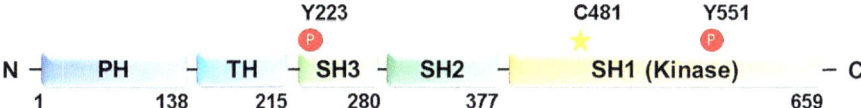

Fig. 2 BTK structure. BTK gene encodes a cytoplasmic protein-tyrosine kinase of 659 amino acids characterized by the following domain organization (from the N-terminus): Pleckstrin homology (PH), Tec homology, SRC homology 3 (SH3), SH2, and catalytic domain (SH1). The position of two tyrosine (Y) phosphorylation sites (Y223 and Y551) and the binding site of ibrutinib (C481) are shown

linemia (Bruton's agammaglobulinemia) [3–5]. The loss of BTK leads to the absence of mature peripheral B cells and very low serum immunoglobulin levels, making affected patients vulnerable to bacterial infections.

Molecular mechanisms leading to this phenotype were elucidated later, understanding that the *BTK* gene encodes a cytoplasmic protein-tyrosine kinase of 659 amino acids characterized by the following domain organization (from the N-terminus): Pleckstrin homology (PH), Tec homology, SRC homology 3 (SH3), SH2, and catalytic domain (SH1) (Fig. 2).

BTK is a member of the TEC kinase family along with TEC (expressed in B-, T-cells and liver cells), ITK (IL2 inducible T-cell kinase), and BMX/ETK (mainly active in bone marrow, endothelia, epithelia).

BTK seems to be required in B cells for BCR-induced calcium release, cell proliferation, and activation of the NF-κB pathway (Fig. 1). The enzyme is also involved in regulating actin dynamics and antigen processing during BCR and promotes B-cell trafficking mediated by the chemokine receptors CXCR4 and CXCR5 [6].

Since BTK is a critical effector molecule for B cell development and lymphomagenesis, BTK inhibitors have been investigated as potential treatments.

The development of BTK inhibitors for use in the treatment of lymphoid malignancies has been rapid during the last decade. In several countries ibrutinib (also known as PCI-32765), the first BTK inhibitor used in clinical trials, has now been approved for the treatment of chronic lymphocytic leukemia (CLL), mantle cell lymphoma (MCL), Waldenström's macroglobulinemia (WM) and Marginal-zone lymphoma (MZL). To date, the use of ibrutinib and second generation BTK-inhibitors (acalabrutinib, CC-292, ONO/GS-4059 and BGB-3111) alone or in different combinations is being explored in a large number of clinical trials.

Following the introduction and use over time of BTK inhibitors the clinical problem of resistance has also arisen, both primary, of particular relevance in MCL, and acquired after longer or shorter periods of time on BTK-inhibitor treatment. Considering that the mechanisms behind resistance also are beginning to be elucidated, it is of interest to review this rapidly progressing field.

As most published data regarding BTK-inhibitor treatment have addressed CLL, this will be the main focus of this review.

Ibrutinib Biochemical Structure, PK, PD, Routes and Doses

Ibrutinib (chemical name 1 [(3R)-3-[4-amino-3-(4-phenoxyphenyl)-1Hpyrazolo[3,4-d]pyrimidin-1-yl]-1-piperidinyl]-2-propen-1-one) is a first-in-class, potent, orally administered covalently-binding inhibitor of BTK.

To date ibrutinib remains the only BTK inhibitor registered for several lymphoproliferative disorders, being approved by the U.S. Food and Drug Administration (FDA) with the following treatment indications:

- patients with mantle cell lymphoma (MCL) who have received at least one prior therapy;
- patients with CLL/small lymphocytic lymphoma (SLL);
- patients with Waldenström's macroglobulinemia (WM)
- patients with marginal zone lymphoma (MZL) who require systemic therapy and have received at least one prior anti-CD20-based therapy. (IMBRUVICA® prescribing information).

Ibrutinib inactivates BTK through an irreversible covalent bond with Cys-481 in the ATP binding domain inhibiting BTK autophosphorylation at tyrosine residue 223 [7].

Inhibition of BTK blocks downstream BcR signaling pathways preventing B-cell proliferation [8], but also interferes with the protective effect of the microenvironment [9]. In vitro, ibrutinib inhibits purified BTK with an IC50 < 10 nM. Selected members of the kinase family with a cysteine residue aligning with Cys481 (including BLK, BMX, ITK, TEC, EGFR, ERBB2 and JAK3) can be covalently bound and inhibited by ibrutinib at concentrations achievable in vivo [10]. Beyond the BCR signaling inhibition, inhibitory effects of ibrutinib on the tumor-microenvironment interactions have been demonstrated, interfering with signals from chemokines, CD40 ligand, BAFF, fibronectin, and TLR ligands [11]. In CLL an impaired homing ability of the leukemic cells, due to reduced chemokine-mediated migration and integrin-dependent adhesion, has been associated with treatment-related lymphocytosis. This "redistribution lymphocytosis" is frequently detected in the first 2 months of treatment in CLL patients, more rarely in lymphoma patients, and in up to 20% of cases may last more than 12 months. In CLL patients the duration of redistribution lymphocytosis seems to be different according to the immunoglobulin gene (IGHV) mutation status, with patients with mutated *IGHV* genes (<98% identity with germline gene, *M-IGHV*) experiencing long-lasting lymphocytosis compared to those with unmutated (≥98% identity with germline gene, *U-IGHV*) IGHV genes. This effect should not be interpreted as sign of progression, if isolated, being frequently linked to a concurrent dramatic and rapid reductions of disease in lymph nodes and the spleen [12, 13].

Intermittent exposure to ibrutinib by once daily administration limits the duration of off-target effects and it is made feasible by the irreversible covalent binding of the compound to BTK [14]. BTK remains fully occupied by ibrutinib for at least 24 h at currently administered dose, despite its rapid clearance from the plasma.

Interestingly, in patients with CLL, the intermittent dosing schedule was associated with transient reversal of treatment-related lymphocytosis during the 7-days-off drug period, suggesting a reversal of the biologic effect [14]. On this basis, and given the tolerability of continuous dosing, the latter was selected for phase II and III studies [15–18].

Ibrutinib is rapidly absorbed, has a high oral plasma clearance (approximately 1000 L/h) and a high apparent volume of distribution at steady state (approximately 10,000 L). Pharmacokinetic (PK) parameters were not dependent on dose, study, or clinical indication [19, 20] The fasting state was characterized by a 67% relative bioavailability compared with the meal conditions used in the trials. Body weight and co-administration of antacids marginally increased the volume of distribution and the duration of absorption, respectively. The linear model indicated that the compound's PK was dose independent and time independent [21].

Ibrutinib is a high hepatic extraction compound whose elimination is predominantly via the CYP3A4 metabolism with minor involvement of CYP2D6. Both CYP3A and CYP2D6 are part of the cytochrome 450 enzymatic machinery in the liver, being the most significant CYP pathways in the oxidative biotransformation of numerous medications. Interactions between ibrutinib and drugs influencing CYP3A4 are of clinical significance [22].

In healthy subjects the co-administration of ibrutinib with ketoconazole (a strong CYP3A inhibitor) increased the maximum serum concentration (Cmax) and area under the curve (AUC) by 29- and 24-fold, respectively. The co-administration of ibrutinib with rifampin (a strong CYP3A inducer) decreased Cmax and AUC by more than 13- and 10-fold, respectively.

Moderate CYP3A4 inhibitors increase ibrutinib exposure 5- to 7-fold, whereas mild CYP3A4 inhibitors were predicted to only marginally increase exposure (about 2-fold) [20]. Moderate CYP3A4 inducers confer a 5- to 7-fold decrease in ibrutinib exposure.

It should also be considered that supplements such as garlic, *Ginkgo biloba*, Echinacea, ginseng, St. John's wort and grape seed alter the exposure of medications metabolized by CYP3A [23]. Patients were excluded from ibrutinib clinical trials if on warfarin and derivatives and/or strong CYP3A inhibitors or inducers while recent analyses in "real-life" setting suggest that 2 out 3 patients treated with ibrutinib in clinical practice are on a concomitant medication with potential to influence ibrutinib metabolism (64% taking concomitant medications with the potential to alter ibrutinib metabolism and/or increase risk of ibrutinib toxicity, 3% on drug potentially reducing ibrutinib efficacy). Further analysis based on clinical practice is thus needed to fully understand the relevance of drug-drug interactions over ibrutinib treatment [24]. Dose reductions are advised in patients with moderate hepatic impairment while the use of ibrutinib in patients with severe hepatic impairment should be avoided because of the risk for excessive exposure/toxicity.

Ibrutinib: Efficacy and Safety Clinical Data

CLL efficacy and safety data In the phase 1 and 1b-2 trials with ibrutinib in patients with relapsed/refractory B-cell malignancies, a maximum tolerated dose (MTD) was not identified and the current dose in CLL (420 mg QD) was defined according to pharmacodynamic parameters. The overall response rate reached 60%, with 13% of CR and a median PFS of 13.6 months. Current registered indication for ibrutinib in CLL derived from the results of two phase 3 trials and one phase 2 trial. The analysis of the RESONATE trial, where ibrutinib monotherapy was compared with ofatumumab single agent in relapsed/refractory CLL documented a clear superiority of ibrutinib, with an ORR of 42.6% (vs 4.1% in the comparison arm, patients with partial response with lymphocytosis were excluded) and a median PFS not yet reached in the ibrutinib arm (in comparison to a median PFS of 8.1 months in the ofatumumab group) [16]. An OS benefit at 12 months was demonstrated in the ibrutinib arm (90% of patients on ibrutinib still alive vs 81% of patients treated with ofatumumab). Adverse events (AEs) of any grade occurring in ≥25% of patients treated with ibrutinib turned out to be diarrhea (mainly grade 1 and 2), upper respiratory tract infection, fatigue, cough, arthralgia, rash, pyrexia and peripheral edema. Rarer AEs, though clinically relevant, include atrial fibrillation and bleeding events.

RESONATE-2 results comparing ibrutinib monotherapy with chlorambucil single-agent in treatment-naïve elderly CLL patients led to the approval by FDA in first-line setting [25]. The ORR in ibrutinib-treated patients was 86% (vs 35% in chlorambucil arm), the PFS not reached and the risk of progression or death was reduced by 84% in patients treated with ibrutinib, leading to an estimated OS rate of 98% with ibrutinib compared to 85% with chlorambucil.

The results of an Ohio State trial, that retrospectively studied 308 patients on ibrutinib treatment, were published in 2015 [26]. After a median follow-up of 20 months, 18 (6%) patients had discontinued treatment due to transformation while 13 (4%) did so due to progression, with the data showing transformation occurring early during treatment while progression occurred later on.

Outside the setting of clinical trials, retrospective data on patients treated within population-based cohorts have recently been published. A population-based Swedish cohort was reported, including 95 consecutive R/R CLL patients treated within a compassionate use program with ORR rate of 84% in a population with two thirds having TP53 aberration [27]. With a follow-up of 10 months was reported 7 (7%) progressive CLL and 3 (3%) with transformation. The UK CLL forum reported data on 315 patients with one third having TP53 aberrations and after a median follow-up of 16.5 months 14 (4.5%) patients with progression as well as 14 patients (4.5%) developing transformation [28].

As treatment with single-agent ibrutinib seldom lead to complete remissions and, as mentioned, a large proportion of patients have a prolonged lymphocytosis [29], different schedules of BTK-inhibitors in combination with chemotherapy, CD20-antibodies and Bcl-2 inhibitors are at the moment being explored in a great number of trials. The rationale behind this is that combination treatments can lead to deeper responses and reduce the risk of clonal evolution in prevailing CLL-cells.

The published data regarding combination treatments are few to date. In 2014 a phase 2 study was published with the combination of ibrutinib + rituximab in a cohort of high-risk CLL patients, reporting an ORR of 97%. An extended analysis of this cohort after a median of 47 months was recently presented in which it was reported 8 patients (20%) with progressive disease and 2 (5%) with Richter's transformation [30].

The results of a phase 3 study (HELIOS trial) reported a significantly longer PFS with the combination of ibrutinib plus bendamustine and rituximab -BR- (estimated PFS at 18 months 79% in the ibrutinib plus BR vs 24% in the placebo plus BR arm) [31]. The minimal residual disease (MRD) negativity rate (a strong positive prognostic indicator correlating with prolonged response duration and survival) in patients treated with the combination of ibrutinib and BR increased after continuing treatment with ibrutinib and reached 20.7%, compared to 1.4% in the BR-plus-placebo group. These results led to the approval of ibrutinib plus BR for relapsed/refractory CLL by FDA. That notwithstanding, the potential benefit of adding immunotherapy or chemoimmunotherapy to ibrutinib single-agent is still under investigation.

MCL efficacy and safety data Ibrutinib has been approved for the treatment of patients with MCL who have received at least 1 prior therapy. The dose in MCL, higher than in CLL, is 560 mg QD. This indication was derived from the results of a phase 2 study in which 111 heavily pretreated R/R MCL patients were treated with ibrutinib 560 mg daily [32]. With 86% of the patients having intermediate/high-risk disease, they were divided into two groups based on previous exposure to bortezomib. The ORR was 68% with 21% being complete responses, with no differences depending on previous bortezomib or not, whereas 32% had stable or progressive disease. Follow-up data after a median follow-up of 26.7 months from this trial reported an ORR of 67% with 23% CR. The median progression-free survival was 13 months with a PFS rate at 24 months of 31% and an OS rate at 24 months of 47% [33].

A second phase 2 trial confirmed these findings, reporting a median PFS of 10.5 months with an OS rate of 61% at 18 months. Common adverse events were diarrhea, fatigue, and nausea while hematologic toxicity was uncommon. Despite the significant efficacy, about one third of patients was primary resistant to ibrutinib treatment and the acquired resistance appeared to eventually occur in all MCL patients. Results of a phase 3 study comparing the efficacy of ibrutinib with temsirolimus in 280 relapsed MCL patients confirmed a prolonged PFS (14.6 vs 6.2 months) and a better tolerability (grade 3 or higher treatment-emergent adverse events 68% vs 87%) in ibrutinib treated group [34]. Of the 139 patients treated with ibrutinib 74 discontinued treatment of whom 55 did so due to disease progression.

WM efficacy and safety data Ibrutinib was approved by the FDA for the treatment of patients with treatment-naïve or relapsed refractory WM, based on the results of a prospective study of ibrutinib monotherapy (at a dose of 420 mg/day) in 63 patients with WM relapsing or refractory after at least one previous treatment [35]. The ORR was 91%, with no complete responses but a major response rate of 73%. The estimated 2-year PFS and OS rates were 69% and 95%, respectively. Notably, the drug showed a favorable toxicity profile with treatment-related hematologic toxicities (grade ≥3) being represented by neutropenia (15%) and thrombocytopenia (13%), mainly in heavily pretreated patients. Non-hematologic toxicities recorded were mild-moderate bleeding events and atrial fibrillation associated with a history of arrhythmia (5%). Similar efficacy results were obtained as part of a larger prospective trial, where ibrutinib monotherapy (at a dose of 420 mg/day) was given in 31 patients with disease refractory to rituximab [36]. The ORR was 84%, including 65% major responses, with PFS and OS analysis still awaited considering the short follow up.

Marginal-zone lymphoma (MZL) efficacy and safety data The results of an open-label, multicenter, phase II trial of ibrutinib in 60 patients with MZL who had received at least one prior therapy were recently reported and led to the FDA approval for relapsed/refractory MZL [37]. After a median follow up of 19.4 months, the ORR was 48% with a median PFS of 14.2 months and a median duration of response not reached. The safety profile confirmed expected treatment-emergent AEs, with anemia (14%), pneumonia (8%), and fatigue (6%) being the most common grade ≥3 events.

Other NHL efficacy and safety data Modest benefit has been documented with ibrutinib single-agent in patients with other B-cell malignancies including follicular lymphoma (FL) and activated B-cell type diffuse large B-cell lymphoma (ABC-DLBCL) [14, 38]. The drug is currently explored in combination with immunotherapy, chemotherapy and novel targeted therapies in these B-cell lymphoproliferative disorders.

Resistance to BTK Inhibitors

With ibrutinib in many instances showing superior efficacy compared to older treatments, and gaining breakthrough designation from the FDA, its use in clinical practice has been widely implemented in a short period of time. Hence, there is still a lack of solid data regarding treatment outcome over a longer time span.

Important to bear in mind is also the fact that CLL, MCL, WM and MZL, the lymphoproliferative disorders for which the drug is approved, differ in disease biology, presentation, treatment options, prognosis, response to treatment with ibrutinib, as well as known resistance mechanisms to the same drug. As a consequence, comparisons between clinical data regarding resistance to treatment among these different diagnoses are difficult to be made.

Also important to take into account when evaluating the published clinical trials regarding the variety of study populations (treatment naïve vs. relapsed/refractory), time of follow-up, dosage of the BTK-inhibitor and risk profile regarding disease biology (*TP53* aberrations, mutational status of the IGHV genes, etc.)

When evaluating resistance, the number of clinical trials reporting the underlying mechanisms are few, but of course of great interest when trying to elucidate the topic. To get a broader picture of the risk for developing resistance to treatment, it is also of use to study the reported number of treatment discontinuations, the number of patients with progressive disease and the number of patients with disease transformation in published clinical trials.

An overview of selected trials with BTK inhibitors in CLL in regard to these parameters is presented in Table 1.

Clinical Studies on Resistance Mechanisms in CLL

As mentioned, mechanisms of resistance are different according to disease biology and still need to be fully elucidated. In CLL, primary resistance (i.e. patients who lack disease control on ibrutinib from the beginning) is a quite infrequent event while secondary resistance does occur over the disease course. Early relapses (within the first 12–24 months) are usually associated with disease transformation (so called Richter' syndrome or prolymphocytic leukemia) while late relapses (>24 months) maintain CLL characteristics.

Since ibrutinib acts as an irreversible inhibitor of BTK and previous experience with hematological malignancies treated with kinase inhibitors suggest that mutations leading to binding site modification are a primary mechanism of resistance, point mutations in key enzymes for BCR signaling have been investigated. Accordingly, BTK and the downstream kinase PLCγ2 mutations were identified in CLL patients progressing on ibrutinib.

In this regard, two seminal papers were published in the New England Journal of Medicine (NEJM) in 2014. Furman et al. described a CLL patient with PR on ibrutinib treatment (560 mg) who after 21 months showed signs of progression [39]. By using sequencing techniques they could find a mutation in BTK (C481S) in samples at time of progression, but not in samples taken before treatment or during response. The substitution of serine for cysteine at residue 481 of BTK (C481S) prevents ibrutinib from covalently binding to the BTK mutants, leading to a reversible inhibition. The IC50 of ibrutinib on C481 mutant BTK was much higher than in the non-mutant form (1006 and 2.2 nM, respectively).

In the same issue of NEJM, Woyach et al. performed whole exome sequencing (WES) in six patients with initial treatment response followed by signs of treatment resistance to ibrutinib [40]. In five of these patients they could find a mutation in BTK (C481S), which they also could show resulting in only reversible inhibition of BTK on functional analysis. In two of the patients, they also found different gain-of-function mutations in PLCγ2 (R665W, S707Y and L845F). As PLCγ2 is

Table 1 Selected trials with BTK inhibitors in CLL

Study	Disease status (treatment-naive or relapsed/refractory)	Number of patients on BTK-inhibitor	Del 17p and/or TP53-mut.0,	U-IGHV	Follow-up time (median)	Treatment	ORR Ibrutinib treated	Treatment discontinuation (in total – due to AE, progression, transformation or other causes)	Progression of CLL (not including transformation)	Transformation
Byrd et al. NEJM 2013 NCT01105247 Phase 1b/2	CLL R/R	85	28 (33%)	69 (81%)	21 months	Ibrutinib 420 mg (n = 51) Ibrutinib 840 mg (n = 34)	89%	31 (36%)	4 (5%)	7 (8%)
O'Brien et al. Lancet Onc. 2014 NCT01105247. Phase 1b/2	CLL TN	31	2 (6%)	15 (48%)	22.1 months	Ibrutinib 420 mg (n = 27) Ibrutinib 840 mg (n = 4)	86%	3 (10%)	1 (3%)	0
Byrd et al. NEJM 2014 NCT01578707 phase 3	CLL R/R	195	63 (32%)	NA	9.4 months	Ibrutinib 420 mg	43% + 20% PR-1	20 (10%)	9 (5%)	3 (1.5%) 2 Richter 1 PLL
Burger et al. NEJM 2015 NCT01722487 phase 3	CLL TN	136	0	58 (43%)	18.4 months	Ibrutinib 420 mg	86%	17 (12.5%)	2 (1.5%)	
Farooqui et al. Blood 2015 NCT01500733 phase 2	CLL TN (n = 35) CLL R/R (n = 16)	51	51 (100%)	22 (63%) + 12 (75%)	15 months +26 months	Ibrutinib 420 mg	97% (untreated) 80% (R/R)	9 (18%)	5 (10%)	3 (3%) Richter 2 (2%) PLL
O'Brien et al. Lancet Onc. 2016 NCT01744691 Phase 2	CLL R/R	144	144 (100%)	97 (67%)	27.6 months (extended analysis)	Ibrutinib 420 mg	83% (extended analysis)	72 (50%)	22 (15%) (extended analysis)	17 (12%)

Study	Population	N			Follow-up	Treatment				
Burger et al. Lancet Onc. 2014 Jain et al. NCT01520519 Phase 2	CLL R/R (n = 36) CLL TN (n = 4)	40	36 (90%)	32 (80%)	16.8 months	Ibrutinib 420 mg + Rituximab	95%	9 (22.5%) 21 (53%) (extended analysis)	2 (5%) 8 (20%) extended follow-up	1 (2.5%) 2 (5%) (extended follow-up)
Chanan-Khan et al. Lancet Onc. 2016 NCT01611090 phase 3	CLL R/R	289	0	210 (81%)	17 months	Ibrutinib 420 mg + Bendamustine+ rituximab	83%	84 (29%)	14 (5%)	0
Byrd et al. Blood 2015 NCT01105247, NCT01109069 follow-up	CLL TN (n = 31) + CLL R/R (n = 101)	132	2 (6%) + 34 (34%)	15 (48%) + 79 (78%)	30 months +23 months	Ibrutinib 420 mg Ibrutinib 840 mg	26 (84%) + 9 (90%)	7 (23%) + 60 (60%) (extended analysis)	1 (1%) +13 (13%) (extended analysis)	8 (6%) (extended analysis)
Maddocks et al. JAMA Onc. 2015 Retrospective NCT01105247, NCT01217749, NCT01589302, NCT01578707	CLL TN (n = 8) CLL R/R (n = 300)	308	113 (37%)	219 (80%)	20 months	Ibrutinib 420 mg Ibrutinib 420 + Ofatumumab	NA	76 (25%)	13 (4%)	18 (6%)
Winqvist et al. Haematologica 2016 Retrospective	CLL R/R	95	63 (66%)	NA	10.2 months	Ibrutinib 420 mg	84%	23 (24%)	7 (7%)	3 (3%)
UK CLL forum Heamatologica 2016 retrospective	CLL R/R	315	90/263 (34.2%)	NA	16 months	Ibrutinib 420 mg	NA	83 (26%)	14 (4.5%)	14 (4.5%)

immediately downstream to BTK, these mutants allow autonomous BCR signaling despite inactive BTK.

Deep-sequencing data on 11 patients with disease progression (3 of which were reported in [40]) and 8 with transformation were published in 2015 by the same group, analyzing pretreatment and relapse samples [26]. They could find BTK-mutations (C481S and C481F) and/or PLCγ2-mutations (R665W, S707P, S707F, S707Y,R742P, D1140G and L845 fs) in all patients. In the 8 patients with transformation they found 1 patient with 3 separate mutations in BTK (C481S, T474I, and T474S), and 1 with 3 separate mutations in BTK (C481Y, C481R, and L528 W) combined with a PLCγ2-mutation (D334H) [26].

Computational evolutionary models have suggested that the development of resistance due to mutations in BTK or PLCγ2 could be a result of selection of microclones during treatment [41], although in the two described papers in NEJM the researchers also performed sequencing of pretreatment samples without findings of these mutations. Furthermore, a recent Italian study examined 613 ibrutinib-naïve CLL-patients without any findings of BTK- or PLCγ2-mutations [42].

Looking further into the question of clonal evolution, in a study published in 2016, Burger et al. analyzed sequential samples from five ibrutinib-treated patients using whole-exome and deep-targeted sequencing [43]. The researchers could find a clonal expansion in three of the patients of clones harboring del8p, postulating this resulting in TRAIL-insensitivity which may lead to ibrutinib resistance. They also demonstrated the presence of pretreatment ibrutinib resistant subclones. In the two other patients they demonstrated a BTK-mutation (C481S) and multiple PLCγ2-mutations.

Complete response (CR) rates in both treatment-naïve (TN) CLL and relapsed/refractory (R/R CLL) on treatment with ibrutinib as a single drug are quite low, thus, reflecting the inherent insensitivity and/or resistance to the drug that occurs in a number of CLL-cells.

That notwithstanding, the clinical impact of this has not yet been clarified as shown by the fact that patients with long-standing lymphocytosis do not seem to have a worse prognosis than those without. Along this line deep-sequencing on nine patients with persistent lymphocytosis (more than 12 months) demonstrated no evidence of either BTK- or PLCγ2-mutations, thus suggesting that peripheral blood CLL cells in these patients constitute a quiescent CLL clone, though resistant to ibrutinib-induced apoptosis.

Risk factors for ibrutinib resistance have not yet been fully addressed, but some factors have been associated with increased risk in different series, including a complex karyotype, *TP53* aberrations and a number of previous therapies.

The published clinical trials on ibrutinib-treated relapsed/refractory CLL, excluding RESONATE-17 which recruited only patients with deletion17p, have a median follow-up of 10–28 months (Table 1). The reported percentage of CLL-progression without transformation amounts to approximately 5% and the number of patients reported to have developed transformation ranges from 1.5% to 8%. Of notice is that the studied populations to a large extent exhibit high-risk features such as multiple lines of treatment, *TP53* aberrations and U-IGHV.

The pivotal phase 3 RESONATE-trial comparing ibrutinib with ofatumumab for R/R CLL reported 195 high-risk CLL patients treated with ibrutinib with a median follow-up of 9.4 months having an ORR of 63% and 5% having progression of CLL and 1.5% developing transformation [16].

Two studies have included patients with *TP53* aberrations [44, 45]. As noted before, this is the subgroup in CLL with historically the worst prognosis, and due to the TP53-aberration an inherent risk of clonal evolution and selection of resistant clones. In the RESONATE-17 trial, it was reported 15% of patients with CLL progression and 12% with transformation after a median follow-up of 27.6 months [44]. In a trial published in Blood in 2015, including both treatment-naïve and R/R patients with *TP53* aberrations but with a shorter follow-up, it was reported progression in 10% and transformation in 5% of the cases [15].

These data underlines the notion that also with BTK-inhibitor treatment the occurrence of *TP53* aberrations confer an increased risk of treatment failure. This also is clearly evident when comparing subgroups of patients with or without *TP53* aberrations in the other clinical trials on ibrutinib in CLL. Also, noteworthy there are differences among trials regarding the number of patients where sequencing data were available regarding *TP53* mutations for those patients being negative for deletion17p on FISH.

Patients with *TP53* aberrations fare worse in clinical trials than patients without this defect. With a *TP53* aberration present, the genomic instability increases, conferring a higher risk of events leading to resistance and/or transformation of the disease [46]. *TP53* aberration is also associated with patients having a complex karyotype [47]. A study from MD Anderson addressed the issue of the impact of complex karyotype on failure on ibrutinib treatment [48]. They retrospectively studied 88 patients treated with ibrutinib where FISH and metaphase karyotyping had been performed pretreatment. They found that the occurrence of a complex karyotype was a stronger predictor for outcome than deletion17p in their material.

Cumulative analyses of single-center cohorts have been recently published and has helped shedding light in mechanisms underlying ibrutinib resistance in CLL patients [49–51]. In a retrospective analysis of 308 patients with generally high-risk features, who received therapy with ibrutinib single-agent (n = 237) or in combination with ofatumumab (n = 71), 44% were still on treatment after a median follow up of 3.4 years, while 4.5% have undergone transplantation or other treatments and 51% have discontinued ibrutinib [50]. The reason for discontinuation in more than half of cases (83 patients) was disease progression with 55 patients experiencing progressive CLL without transformation. Samples at relapse were tested and in 85% of cases showed the presence of BTK and/or PLCγ2 mutations. With retrospective serial sampling evaluation, a clone of resistant CLL-cells could be identified up to 18 months before clinical relapse (median time 9.3 months).

In 112 CLL patients on ibrutinib followed at the same institution the occurrence of BTK and PLCγ2 mutations was prospectively evaluated. Of the eight patients experiencing clinical relapse all had a C481S BTK mutation detectable. The mutation was present also in samples collected before relapse. Eight additional cases showed the presence of the same mutation without meeting the criteria for clinical relapse.

More than 1200 samples from 373 CLL patients from The Ohio State University (OSU) were sequenced for BTK and PLCγ2 coding [49]. Up to 23.3% of patients showed BTK mutations in codon 481 with above 1% variant allele frequency (VAF) in at least one sample and up to 9.7% of the patients showed recurrent/hotspot PLCγ2 mutations. The detection of PLCγ2 mutations was clearly associated with BTK mutation occurrence and suggests a multistep resistance pattern. Interestingly enough, an additional hotspot for resistance-associated mutations was identified in the C2 domain of the protein, potentially leading to a complex regulatory shift in the PLCγ2 protein.

Similar results were obtained in a single-institution trial when analyzing the clinical and molecular characteristics of progressive disease in 84 CLL-patients on single-agent ibrutinib over a median time of 3 years. In this cohort almost 18% of patients progressed, with progressive cases showing a higher prevalence of del(17p), increased β-2 microglobulin, and relapsed or refractory disease [51]. In 60% of progressive cases, the reason for progression was increasing nodal disease. In most cases, ibrutinib-resistant CLL harbored several subclonal mutations involving BTK and/or PLCγ2 characterized by a different growth rate. This finding supports the notion that the clonal complexity is associated with ibrutinib resistance.

It is worth noting that, although mutations in BTK and/or PLCγ2 are found in 85–90% of patients at relapse through high sensitivity assays, they are frequently present in a small percentage of clonal cells. Recently, it has been suggested that circulating CLL cells might not be the most reliable source for testing for these mutations, while testing cell-free DNA (cfDNA) from plasma or serum might provide greater sensitivity, reflecting the whole clonal mutation burden [52].

Risk of progression on ibrutinib is higher in R/R CLL patients compared to TN and in a meta-analysis a relevant reduction in PFS has been reported in patients receiving ibrutinib after >2 lines of treatment. Along this line, published prospective trials with ibrutinib in TN CLL report data with a significantly lower risk of progression than in the R/R group, in the TN patients ranging from 1.5% to 3% with a median follow-up between 18 and 22 months (Table 1).

In the thus far follow-up publications, it was reported extended 44-month follow-up of data [53] from two trials with both TN and R/R CLL-patients [15, 54]. In this publication the reported percentage of CLL progression was 4% and 16% in the two groups respectively, with a total of 3% of patients having disease transformation. This again highlightes the difference in risk between treatment-naïve and previously treated patients. Also of notice is the reported total of 19% TN- and 40% R/R-patients who have discontinued treatment for whatever reason.

Prognosis After Disease Progression and Transformation in CLL

To try to answer the question how patients who discontinued treatment on ibrutinib fare, several retrospective analyses have been published.

In the trial from Ohio, prognosis after stopping ibrutinib for the patients with transformation was dismal, with a median survival of just 3.5 months while the median survival of the patients with CLL progression was 17.6 months, with 2 of them not being fit for more treatment, and 11 being in need of quick retreatment after ibrutinib discontinuation due to rapid progression [26].

The same year a retrospective analysis from MD Anderson studied 33 patients (out of 127) treated with single ibrutinib or in combination with rituximab in various trials and then discontinuing treatment [55]. The patients had an abundance of high-risk features, early progression (within 30 months) and a dismal prognosis, with a median overall survival of 3.1 months after discontinuation. Of these 33 patients 7 discontinued treatment due to progression of CLL and 7 due to transformation. Of the ones with progression 4 out of 7 were alive, and in the transformed group only 1 out of 7 were alive at the time of follow-up.

Recently, a retrospective analysis was published in which 178 patients discontinued treatment with BCR inhibitors (143 ibrutinib and 35 idelalisib) [56]. This also being a high-risk cohort with a median of three previous treatments, deletion17p in 34%, *TP53* mutation in 27% and complex karyotype in 29%. In the ibrutinib-treated cohort 40 (28%) stopped treatment due to progression of CLL and 11 (8%) due to transformation. Of the 114 patients receiving subsequent therapy in both groups the ORR was 50% and PFS 11.9 months. The study also addressed the issue of alternate BCR-inhibitor treatment, showing that the cause of discontinuation is important, with the patients retreated with another BCR inhibitor stopping treatment due to intolerance not having reached median PFS and those stopping due to progression had a median PFS of 7 months.

Resistance Mechanisms in MCL

Although ibrutinib is an effective treatment option in MCL compared to previous treatments, still a significant number of patients are primary resistant to the treatment, exhibiting stable disease or progression on treatment.

The mechanisms behind the primary resistance to ibrutinib in MCL are in most cases to be elucidated. The occurrence of the BTK-mutation C481S as seen in CLL has also been found in MCL but is not the sole explanation [57]. In 2014, Rahal et al. described mechanisms of inherent resistance to ibrutinib through mutations leading to the activation of the alternative NFκB-pathway [58]. Using targeted sequencing on 165 samples from MCL patients they found 6% having TRAF2-mutations and 10% with BIRC3-mutations, both important for NIK-stability and activation of the alternative NFκB-pathway. In vitro studies supported a role for PI3K/AKT activation in determining the response to BTK inhibition in primary MCL cells exposed to ibrutinib. ERK or AKT phosphorylation inhibition showed a linear correlation with the cellular death response caused by ibrutinib, with pERK or pAKT downregulation being associated with ibrutinib response.

Along the same line, recent analyses of de novo and acquired ibrutinib resistance in MCL identified the tumor microenvironment (TME)-mediated interactions as a key factor leading to kinome reprogramming and reciprocal activation of PI3K-AKT-mTOR, and integrin-β1 signaling [59]. PI3K-AKT-mTOR signaling turned out to be a central signaling hub in ibrutinib-resistant MCL cells and high AKT phosphorylation was detected in ibrutinib-resistant MCL cells in the presence of ibrutinib. Ibrutinib resistance did also correlate with increased β1 expression which was involved in functional regulation of the mTORC2-AKT pathway activation, reinforcing TME-lymphoma interactions and promoting MCL growth and drug resistance.

In addition to trials using ibrutinib as a single agent in MCL, several phase 1–2 trials have been published on combination-treatment on both treatment-naïve and relapsed/refractory MCL with different agents (Rituximab, Ublituximab, BR, R-CHOP and Lenalidomide) with ORR reported ranging from 83% to 94% [60]. Several other combinations are also currently being tested in clinical trials.

The prognosis for patients with MCL who are primary resistant or relapse on ibrutinib treatment is dismal. In a retrospective multicenter study, Martin et al. studied 114 patients with MCL with relapse or progression on ibrutinib treatment. Fifty two percentage of the patients were intermediate- or high-risk according to MIPI and the median time on ibrutinib was 4.7 months. After discontinuation of ibrutinib the median overall survival was 2.9 months and the researchers could not identify any post-ibrutinib treatment that was preferable in this setting [61].

Clinical Trials and Resistance Mechanisms in Waldenström's Macroglobulinemia

With Waldenström's macroglobulinemia being characterized by a high frequency (>90%) of the patients displaying a gain-of-function mutation in MYD88 (L265P) leading to BTK- and NFκB-activation [62], much attention regarding the sensitivity to BTK-inhibition has been drawn to the mutational status of MYD88 also in combination with mutations of CXCR4 (WHIM) which is found mutated in about one third of the patients.

In a phase 2 study published in 2015 [63], 63 patients received treatment with ibrutinib in a dose of 420 mg daily with a median duration of treatment being 19.1 months, 78% of patients being intermediate- or high-risk according to IPSSWM and the median number of previous treatments being two.

Interestingly the response-rates differed significantly depending on the mutational status of MYD88/CXCR4. In patients with MYD88^{L265p}/CXCR4^{wt} the ORR was 100% with 91% being major responses, while in patients with MYD88^{L265p} / CXCR4^{whim} the numbers where 86% and 62% and in the cohort with MYD88^{wt}/ CXCR4^{wt} the response rates where down to 71% and 29% respectively. This clearly indicated the role of these mutations in resistance to ibrutinib treatment and giving further evidence of the protective role of the microenvironment in the bone marrow and lymphatic tissues in these diseases.

Recently, CD19+ lymphoplasmacytic cells derived from 6 patients with WM who progressed after achieving major responses on ibrutinib have been sequenced using Sanger sequencing, and detected mutations were validated by targeted next-generation sequencing. Three out of 6 progressive cases showed the presence of BTK C481 variants, including C481S and C481R. In two cases, multiple BTK mutations were detected, showing highly variable clonal distribution. Four out of 5 mutated cases carried CXCR4 mutations before starting ibrutinib [64].

Other BTK Inhibitors

With ibrutinib available in clinical practice and long-term follow-up results from patients enrolled in clinical trials, the most relevant drawbacks becoming evident are represented by the emerging resistance to the drug and the off-target effect of ibrutinib on other kinases, deemed to be responsible for treatment-emergent adverse events. These shortcomings have led to current clinical development of second-generation and more specific BTK inhibitors, such as ACP-196, ONO/GS-4059, BGB-3111, and CC-292.

Acalabrutinib This drug is a novel irreversible second-generation BTK inhibitor that was rationally designed to be more potent and selective than ibrutinib. It binds covalently to Cys481 showing an improved selectivity and in vivo target coverage in comparison to ibrutinib, without inhibiting EGFR, ITK, or TEC. A mouse thrombosis model documented thrombus formation comparable to untreated mice in mice receiving acalabrutinib, while ibrutinib administration led to impaired thrombus formation. This is expected to be associated with reduced bleeding events in clinical trials. The results published so far seem to support this conclusion, with headache, diarrhea, and weight gain being reported as the most common adverse events with acalabrutinib. No Richter's transformation or atrial fibrillation were reported. A phase 1–2, multicenter trial on acalabrutinib was published in NEJM 2016 in which patients were treated with 100–400 mg daily in the phase 1 part and 100 mg twice daily in the phase 2 part [65]. The patients were R/R CLL with a median of 3 previous treatments and with 31% having deletion17p and 75% with U-IGHV. After a median follow-up of 14.3 months, the ORR was 95% (PR 85%, PR with lymphocytosis 10%). The remaining 5% of patients obtained a SD. The patient with progression showed BTK mutation (C481S) in the major clone and mutation in PLCγ2 (L845F) in a minor clone. Results in patients with Richter's transformation have been recently reported and, though preliminary, showed an ORR of 38%, with 14% CR [65].

ONO/GS4059 Is a highly potent and more specific BTK inhibitor, with efficacy that has been documented at preclinical level in ABC-DLBCL cell line (TMD-8) xenograft model. A phase 1 multicenter dose-escalation study (20–600 mg) with ONO/GS-4049 was published in January 2016 [66]. It included 25 patients with R/R CLL of which the researchers reported response to treatment in 24 patients after a median of 80 weeks on treatment, with 21 of them remaining on treatment at the time of the report. Objective responses were documented in 96% of CLL, 92% of MCL, 35% of non-GCB DLBCL patients. The BTK occupancy in the peripheral blood was maintained for at least 24 h across all dose levels and the drug was well tolerated in all groups, without a MTD reached in the CLL group, while in lymphoma cohort 480 mg once daily was defined as the MTD [33].

BGB-3111 Is a more selective BTK inhibitor with superior oral bioavailability, higher BTK specificity than ibrutinib. In recently updated results in CLL patients BGB-3111 was well tolerated, with the most frequent AEs of any attribution being petechiae/ bruising (38%), upper respiratory tract infection (31%), diarrhea (28%), fatigue (24%), and cough (21%), all Grade 1/2, except for 1 grade 3 bleeding events. Grade 2 atrial fibrillation occurred in one pt. After a median follow-up of 7.5 months, the ORR was 90% (PR 79%, PR-L 10%), SD in 7%, 1 patient not evaluable for response. Similar impressive ORR with a favorable tolerability profile have been obtained in relapsed/refractory WM, where the ORR were recently reported to reach 92%, with 83% major responses (33% very good partial response, VGPR, i.e. >90% reduction in IgM and reduction in extramedullary disease and 50% PR, i.e. 50–90% reduction in IgM and reduction in extramedullary disease) [67–69].

CC-292 The first published clinical data on CC-292 was the phase 1 dose-finding study including 113 patients, of which 84 had R/R CLL or SLL receiving the drug in doses ranging from 125 to 1000 mg. In the CLL/SLL cohort the median of prior therapies was 3, with 24% having deletion17p and 54% U-IGHV. The researchers reported treatment discontinuation in 45 out of 84 CLL/SLL-patients (54%) after a median follow-up of 13.4 months [70].

Conclusion

Clinical studies on BTK-inhibitors (mainly ibrutinib) have given relevant insights into resistance mechanisms to treatment by findings of BTK mutations and PLCγ2 mutations in CLL and BTK mutations in MCL, while the mutational pattern of MYD88 and CXCR4 has shown significance in Waldenström's macroglobulinemia. Also evident is the negative impact of *TP53* aberrations and complex karyotypes on the outcome of treatment. Clinical data also point to the fact that previously treated patients, often having an accumulation of traditional risk-factors, have a higher risk for progression and transformation in comparison to treatment-naïve patients. Currently available data indicate the risk for the latter group to progress or transform on BTK-inhibitor treatment to be low although longer follow-up needs to be done.

The resistance mechanisms seem to differ among different lymphoproliferative malignancies which also is evident in the clinical setting with for example CLL having very few primary resistant cases, in contrary to MCL where this is quite a common event.

At present, data from trials regarding the impact of combination of BTK-inhibitors with other treatments is still too scarce to draw any conclusions and the same applies to the impact of second generation BTK inhibitors.

Further work needs to be done to elucidate the mechanisms behind primary refractory patients, to define the risk for clonal evolution/new mutations over time on treatment, and to identify prognostic/predictive markers for patients on BTK inhibitors.

Acknowledgements The Authors would like to thank Dr. Panagiotis Baliakas for his critical review of the manuscript and his helpful suggestions.

References

1. Gauld SB, Dal Porto JM, Cambier JCB. Cell antigen receptor signaling: roles in cell development and disease. Science. 2002;296:1641–2.
2. Dal Porto JM, Gauld SB, Merrell KT, Mills D, Pugh-Bernard AE, Cambier JB. Cell antigen receptor signaling 101. Mol Immunol. 2004;41:599–613.
3. Bruton OC. Agammaglobulinemia. Pediatrics. 1952;9:722–8.
4. Naor D, Bentwich Z, Cividalli G. Inability of peripheral lymphoid cells of agammaglobulinaemic patients to bind radioiodinated albumins. Aust J Exp Biol Med Sci. 1969;47:759–61.
5. Cooper MD, Lawton AR, Bockman DE. Agammaglobulinaemia with B lymphocytes. Specific defect of plasma-cell differentiation. Lancet. 1971;2:791–4.
6. Niemann CU, Wiestner A. B-cell receptor signaling as a driver of lymphoma development and evolution. Semin Cancer Biol. 2013;23:410–21.
7. Singh J, Petter RC, Kluge AF. Targeted covalent drugs of the kinase family. Curr Opin Chem Biol. 2010;14:475–80.
8. Wiestner A. BCR pathway inhibition as therapy for chronic lymphocytic leukemia and lymphoplasmacytic lymphoma. Hematology Am Soc Hematol Educ Program. 2014;2014:125–34.
9. Spaargaren M, Beuling EA, Rurup ML, et al. The B cell antigen receptor controls integrin activity through Btk and PLCgamma2. J Exp Med. 2003;198:1539–50.
10. Honigberg LA, Smith AM, Sirisawad M, et al. The Bruton tyrosine kinase inhibitor PCI-32765 blocks B-cell activation and is efficacious in models of autoimmune disease and B-cell malignancy. Proc Natl Acad Sci U S A. 2010;107:13075–80.
11. Wiestner A. The role of B-cell receptor inhibitors in the treatment of patients with chronic lymphocytic leukemia. Haematologica. 2015;100:1495–507.
12. Herman SE, Niemann CU, Farooqui M, et al. Ibrutinib-induced lymphocytosis in patients with chronic lymphocytic leukemia: correlative analyses from a phase II study. Leukemia. 2014;28:2188–96.
13. Cheson BD, Byrd JC, Rai KR, et al. Novel targeted agents and the need to refine clinical end points in chronic lymphocytic leukemia. J Clin Oncol. 2012;30:2820–2.
14. Advani RH, Buggy JJ, Sharman JP, et al. Bruton tyrosine kinase inhibitor ibrutinib (PCI-32765) has significant activity in patients with relapsed/refractory B-cell malignancies. J Clin Oncol. 2013;31:88–94.
15. Byrd JC, Furman RR, Coutre SE, et al. Targeting BTK with ibrutinib in relapsed chronic lymphocytic leukemia. N Engl J Med. 2013;369:32–42.
16. Byrd JC, Brown JR, O'Brien S, et al. Ibrutinib versus ofatumumab in previously treated chronic lymphoid leukemia. N Engl J Med. 2014;371:213–23.

17. Byrd JC, Furman RR, Coutre SE, et al. Three-year follow-up of treatment-naive and previously treated patients with CLL and SLL receiving single-agent ibrutinib. Blood. 2015;125:2497–506.
18. Burger JA, Styles L, Kipps TJ. Ibrutinib for chronic lymphocytic leukemia. N Engl J Med. 2016;374:1594–5.
19. Scheers E, Leclercq L, de Jong J, et al. Absorption, metabolism, and excretion of oral (1)(4)C radiolabeled ibrutinib: an open-label, phase I, single-dose study in healthy men. Drug Metab Dispos. 2015;43:289–97.
20. Waldron M, Winter A, Hill BT. Pharmacokinetic and Pharmacodynamic considerations in the treatment of chronic lymphocytic leukemia: Ibrutinib, Idelalisib, and Venetoclax. Clin Pharmacokinet. 2017;56:1255–66.
21. Marostica E, Sukbuntherng J, Loury D, et al. Population pharmacokinetic model of ibrutinib, a Bruton tyrosine kinase inhibitor, in patients with B cell malignancies. Cancer Chemother Pharmacol. 2015;75:111–21.
22. de Zwart L, Snoeys J, De Jong J, Sukbuntherng J, Mannaert E, Monshouwer M. Ibrutinib dosing strategies based on interaction potential of CYP3A4 perpetrators using physiologically based pharmacokinetic modeling. Clin Pharmacol Ther. 2016;100:548–57.
23. de Vries R, Smit JW, Hellemans P, et al. Stable isotope-labelled intravenous microdose for absolute bioavailability and effect of grapefruit juice on ibrutinib in healthy adults. Br J Clin Pharmacol. 2016;81:235–45.
24. Finnes HD, Chaffee KG, Call TG, et al. Pharmacovigilance during ibrutinib therapy for chronic lymphocytic leukemia (CLL)/small lymphocytic lymphoma (SLL) in routine clinical practice. Leuk Lymphoma. 2017;58:1376–83.
25. Burger JA, Tedeschi A, Barr PM, et al. Ibrutinib as initial therapy for patients with chronic lymphocytic leukemia. N Engl J Med. 2015;373:2425–37.
26. Maddocks KJ, Ruppert AS, Lozanski G, et al. Etiology of Ibrutinib therapy discontinuation and outcomes in patients with chronic lymphocytic leukemia. JAMA Oncol. 2015;1:80–7.
27. Winqvist M, Asklid A, Andersson PO, et al. Real-world results of ibrutinib in patients with relapsed or refractory chronic lymphocytic leukemia: data from 95 consecutive patients treated in a compassionate use program. A study from the Swedish chronic lymphocytic leukemia group. Haematologica. 2016;101:1573–80.
28. Ibrutinib for relapsed/refractory chronic lymphocytic leukemia: a UK and Ireland analysis of outcomes in 315 patients. Haematologica. 2016;101:1563–72.
29. Woyach JA, Smucker K, Smith LL, et al. Prolonged lymphocytosis during ibrutinib therapy is associated with distinct molecular characteristics and does not indicate a suboptimal response to therapy. Blood. 2014;123:1810–7.
30. Jain P, Keating MJ, Wierda WG, et al. Long-term follow-up of treatment with Ibrutinib and rituximab in patients with high-risk chronic lymphocytic leukemia. Clin Cancer Res. 2016; 23(9): 2154–58.
31. Chanan-Khan A, Cramer P, Demirkan F, et al. Ibrutinib combined with bendamustine and rituximab compared with placebo, bendamustine, and rituximab for previously treated chronic lymphocytic leukaemia or small lymphocytic lymphoma (HELIOS): a randomised, double-blind, phase 3 study. Lancet Oncol. 2016;17:200–11.
32. Wang ML, Rule S, Martin P, et al. Targeting BTK with ibrutinib in relapsed or refractory mantle-cell lymphoma. N Engl J Med. 2013;369:507–16.
33. Wang ML, Blum KA, Martin P, et al. Long-term follow-up of MCL patients treated with single-agent ibrutinib: updated safety and efficacy results. Blood. 2015;126:739–45.
34. Dreyling M, Jurczak W, Jerkeman M, et al. Ibrutinib versus temsirolimus in patients with relapsed or refractory mantle-cell lymphoma: an international, randomized, open-label, phase 3 study. Lancet. 2016;387:770–8.
35. Treon SP, Tripsas CK, Meid K, et al. Ibrutinib in previously treated Waldenstrom's macroglobulinemia. N Engl J Med. 2015;372:1430–40.
36. Dimopoulos MA, Trotman J, Tedeschi A, et al. Ibrutinib for patients with rituximab-refractory Waldenstrom's macroglobulinaemia (iNNOVATE): an open-label substudy of an international, multicentre, phase 3 trial. Lancet Oncol. 2017;18:241–50.

37. Noy A, de Vos S, Thieblemont C, et al. Targeting Bruton tyrosine kinase with ibrutinib in relapsed/refractory marginal zone lymphoma. Blood. 2017;129:2224–32.
38. Wilson WH, Young RM, Schmitz R, et al. Targeting B cell receptor signaling with ibrutinib in diffuse large B cell lymphoma. Nat Med. 2015;21:922–6.
39. Furman RR, Cheng S, Lu P, et al. Ibrutinib resistance in chronic lymphocytic leukemia. N Engl J Med. 2014;370:2352–4.
40. Woyach JA, Furman RR, Liu TM, et al. Resistance mechanisms for the Bruton's tyrosine kinase inhibitor ibrutinib. N Engl J Med. 2014;370:2286–94.
41. Komarova NL, Burger JA, Wodarz D. Evolution of ibrutinib resistance in chronic lymphocytic leukemia (CLL). Proc Natl Acad Sci U S A. 2014;111:13906–11.
42. Fama R, Bomben R, Rasi S, et al. Ibrutinib-naive chronic lymphocytic leukemia lacks Bruton tyrosine kinase mutations associated with treatment resistance. Blood. 2014;124:3831–3.
43. Burger JA, Landau DA, Taylor-Weiner A, et al. Clonal evolution in patients with chronic lymphocytic leukaemia developing resistance to BTK inhibition. Nat Commun. 2016;7:11589.
44. O'Brien S, Jones JA, Coutre SE, et al. Ibrutinib for patients with relapsed or refractory chronic lymphocytic leukaemia with 17p deletion (RESONATE-17): a phase 2, open-label, multicentre study. Lancet Oncol. 2016;17:1409–18.
45. Farooqui MZ, Valdez J, Martyr S, et al. Ibrutinib for previously untreated and relapsed or refractory chronic lymphocytic leukaemia with TP53 aberrations: a phase 2, single-arm trial. Lancet Oncol. 2015;16:169–76.
46. Te Raa GD, Kater AP. TP53 dysfunction in CLL: implications for prognosis and treatment. Best Pract Res Clin Haematol. 2016;29:90–9.
47. Blanco G, Puiggros A, Baliakas P, et al. Karyotypic complexity rather than chromosome 8 abnormalities aggravates the outcome of chronic lymphocytic leukemia patients with TP53 aberrations. Oncotarget. 2016;7:80916–24.
48. Thompson PA, O'Brien SM, Wierda WG, et al. Complex karyotype is a stronger predictor than del(17p) for an inferior outcome in relapsed or refractory chronic lymphocytic leukemia patients treated with ibrutinib-based regimens. Cancer. 2015;121:3612–21.
49. Jones D, Woyach JA, Zhao W, et al. PLCG2 C2 domain mutations co-occur with BTK and PLCG2 resistance mutations in chronic lymphocytic leukemia undergoing ibrutinib treatment. Leukemia. 2017;31:1645–7.
50. Woyach JA, Ruppert AS, Guinn D, et al. BTKC481S-mediated resistance to Ibrutinib in chronic lymphocytic leukemia. J Clin Oncol. 2017;35(13):1437–43. JCO2016702282.
51. Ahn IE, Underbayev C, Albitar A, et al. Clonal evolution leading to ibrutinib resistance in chronic lymphocytic leukemia. Blood. 2017;129:1469–79.
52. Albitar A, Ma W, DeDios I, et al. Using high-sensitivity sequencing for the detection of mutations in BTK and PLC gamma 2 genes in cellular and cell-free DNA and correlation with progression in patients treated with BTK inhibitors. Oncotarget. 2017;8:17936–44.
53. Coutre SE, Furman RR, Flinn IW, et al. Extended treatment with single-agent Ibrutinib at the 420 mg dose leads to durable responses in chronic lymphocytic leukemia/small lymphocytic lymphoma. Clin Cancer Res. 2017;23:1149–55.
54. O'Brien S, Furman RR, Coutre SE, et al. Ibrutinib as initial therapy for elderly patients with chronic lymphocytic leukaemia or small lymphocytic lymphoma: an open-label, multicentre, phase 1b/2 trial. Lancet Oncol. 2014;15:48–58.
55. Jain P, Keating M, Wierda W, et al. Outcomes of patients with chronic lymphocytic leukemia after discontinuing ibrutinib. Blood. 2015;125:2062–7.
56. Mato AR, Nabhan C, Barr PM, et al. Outcomes of CLL patients treated with sequential kinase inhibitor therapy: a real world experience. Blood. 2016;128:2199–205.
57. Chiron D, Di Liberto M, Martin P, et al. Cell-cycle reprogramming for PI3K inhibition overrides a relapse-specific C481S BTK mutation revealed by longitudinal functional genomics in mantle cell lymphoma. Cancer Discov. 2014;4:1022–35.
58. Rahal R, Frick M, Romero R, et al. Pharmacological and genomic profiling identifies NF-kappaB-targeted treatment strategies for mantle cell lymphoma. Nat Med. 2014;20:87–92.
59. Zhao X, Lwin T, Silva A, et al. Unification of de novo and acquired ibrutinib resistance in mantle cell lymphoma. Nat Commun. 2017;8:14920.

60. Stephens DM, Spurgeon SE. Ibrutinib in mantle cell lymphoma patients: glass half full? evidence and opinion. Ther Adv Hematol. 2015;6:242–52.
61. Martin P, Maddocks K, Leonard JP, et al. Postibrutinib outcomes in patients with mantle cell lymphoma. Blood. 2016;127:1559–63.
62. Treon SP, Xu L, Yang G, et al. MYD88 L265P somatic mutation in Waldenstrom's macroglobulinemia. N Engl J Med. 2012;367:826–33.
63. Treon SP, Xu L, Hunter Z. MYD88 mutations and response to Ibrutinib in Waldenstrom's Macroglobulinemia. N Engl J Med. 2015;373(6):584.
64. Xu L, Tsakmaklis N, Yang G, et al. Acquired mutations associated with ibrutinib resistance in Waldenstrom Macroglobulinemia. Blood. 2017;129(18):2519–25.
65. Byrd JC, Harrington B, O'Brien S, et al. Acalabrutinib (ACP-196) in relapsed chronic lymphocytic leukemia. N Engl J Med. 2016;374:323–32.
66. Walter HS, Rule SA, Dyer MJ, et al. A phase 1 clinical trial of the selective BTK inhibitor ONO/GS-4059 in relapsed and refractory mature B-cell malignancies. Blood. 2016;127:411–9.
67. Wu J, Liu C, Tsui ST, Liu D. Second-generation inhibitors of Bruton tyrosine kinase. J Hematol Oncol. 2016;9:80.
68. Tam CS, Opat S, Cull G, et al. Twice daily dosing with the highly specific BTK inhibitor, Bgb-3111, achieves complete and continuous BTK occupancy in lymph nodes, and is associated with durable responses in patients (pts) with chronic lymphocytic leukemia (CLL)/small lymphocytic lymphoma (SLL). Blood. 2016;128: 642.
69. Tam CS, Trotman J, Opat S, et al. High major response rate, including very good partial responses (VGPR), in patients (pts) with Waldenstrom Macroglobulinemia (WM) treated with the high-ly specific BTK inhibitor Bgb-3111: expansion phase results from an ongoing phase I study. Blood. 2016;128: 1216.
70. Brown JR, Harb WA, Hill BT, et al. Phase I study of single-agent CC-292, a highly selective Bruton's tyrosine kinase inhibitor, in relapsed/refractory chronic lymphocytic leukemia. Haematologica. 2016;101:e295–8.

BCL2 Inhibitors: Insights into Resistance

Mary Ann Anderson, Andrew W. Roberts, and John F. Seymour

Abstract Over the last decade, improved understanding of the mechanisms and structures of proteins integral to apoptosis have enabled therapeutic targeting of BCL2 to become more specific, less toxic and ultimately more clinically effective. The first BCL2-selective inhibitor, venetoclax, is now approved for use in patients with relapsed and refractory chronic lymphocytic leukemia (CLL) in multiple countries. Early phase clinical trials demonstrated an 80% overall response rates in patients with relapsed/refractory CLL, independent of traditional risk factors, without undue toxicity. Venetoclax is also highly active in other lymphoid malignancies that express high levels of its target, BCL2, such as mantle cell lymphoma. However, there is a cumulative incidence of disease progression while on therapy. Ongoing follow-up of the early phase trials is only now enabling elucidation of the incidence and risk factors for disease progression and treatment failure. Preventing development of resistance to BCL2 inhibition requires further research aimed at delineating

M. A. Anderson
Department of Haematology, Royal Melbourne Hospital & Peter MacCallum Cancer Centre, Parkville, VIC, Australia

Division of Cancer and Haematology, Walter and Eliza Hall Institute, Parkville, VIC, Australia

A. W. Roberts
Department of Haematology, Royal Melbourne Hospital & Peter MacCallum Cancer Centre, Parkville, VIC, Australia

Division of Cancer and Haematology, Walter and Eliza Hall Institute, Parkville, VIC, Australia

The University of Melbourne, Melbourne, VIC, Australia

J. F. Seymour (✉)
Department of Haematology, Royal Melbourne Hospital & Peter MacCallum Cancer Centre, Parkville, VIC, Australia

The University of Melbourne, Melbourne, VIC, Australia
e-mail: john.seymour@petermac.org

© Springer International Publishing AG, part of Springer Nature 2018
A. J. M. Ferreri (ed.), *Resistance of Targeted Therapies Excluding Antibodies for Lymphomas*, Resistance to Targeted Anti-Cancer Therapeutics 17,
https://doi.org/10.1007/978-3-319-75184-9_2

the genetic and epigenetic drivers of disease progression. This will facilitate targeting of resistance mechanisms through the use of rational drug combinations, help to prospectively identify patients most likely to benefit and abet early identification of emerging resistance. These therapies are improving outcomes for patients with previously poor prognosis disease.

Keywords BCL2 (B cell lymphoma 2) · Apoptosis · Venetoclax · Chronic lymphocytic leukemia

Abbreviations

AML	Acute myeloid leukemia
BCL2	B cell lymphoma 2
BCR	B cell receptor
BH	BCL2 homology
BTK	Burtons tyrosine kinase
CI	Confidence interval
CLL	Chronic lymphocytic leukemia
CR	Complete remission
CRi	Complete remission, incomplete count recovery
Del11q	Deletion 11q
Del17p	Deletion 17p
DLBCL	Diffuse large B cell lymphoma
DLT	Dose limiting toxicity
DOR	Duration of response
EC_{50}	Half maximal effective concentration
EFS	Event free survival
FFP	Freedom from progression
FL	Follicular lymphoma
G	Grade
HL	Hodgkin lymphoma
IDH	Isocitrate dehydrogenase
IGVH	Immunoglobulin variable region heavy chain
IHC	Immunohistochemistry
MCL	Mantle cell lymphoma
MLL	Mixed lineage leukemia
MM	Multiple myeloma
MRD	Minimal residual disease
MTD	Maximum tolerated dose
MZL	Marginal zone lymphoma
NA	Not applicable
NHL	Non-Hodgkin lymphoma
nM	Nano-molar

ORR	Overall response rate
OS	Overall survival
PD	Progressive disease
PFS	Progression free survival
PI3κ	Phosphoinositide 3 kinase
PR	Partial response
RP2D	Recommended phase 2 dose
RT	Richter's transformation
SLL	Small lymphocytic lymphoma
TLS	Tumor lysis syndrome
TTP	Time to progression
WM	Waldenstrom's macroglobulinemia

Introduction

The advent of rituximab and other monoclonal antibodies, in combination with standard cytotoxic chemotherapy, have heralded a new era of durable remissions in many challenging B cell lymphomas and leukemias [1, 2]. Chronic lymphocytic leukemia (CLL) is the most common adult leukemia in Western countries and is traditionally considered an indolent disorder. Together deletion 17p (del17p) and deletion 11 q (del11q) CLL account for approximately 25% of patients and these individuals have a significantly inferior survival [3]. Other patients whose disease falls into a high-risk category include patients with complex cytogenetics [4], bulky nodal disease [5, 6], fludarabine refractory disease [5–9], and unmutated immunoglobulin variable heavy chain (*IGVH*) gene [10]. For such patients, approaches other than traditional chemo-immunotherapy are required due to the low probability of durable responses.

The last 5 years have seen the emergence of a number of novel targeted agents, for instance the Brutons' tyrosine kinase inhibitor (BTKi), ibrutinib, and the phosphoinositide 3 kinase (PI3κ) inhibitor, idelalisib. Both these agents achieve high response rates in relapsed and refractory CLL. However, the longer term durability of response varies [11, 12], and not all patients are able to tolerate chronic administration of these drugs [13, 14].

Another promising novel approach to treatment in non-Hodgkin lymphoma (NHL) and CLL is to enhance malignant cell death through therapeutic manipulation of the intrinsic pathway of apoptosis. While the concept of targeting this pathway is not new, it is only in recent years that specific and potent agents acting on this pathway have become available. To date the most promising of these is venetoclax, which entered clinical trials in 2011. This review examines its mechanism of action, summarizes key clinical data and explores emerging data about how resistance can emerge.

BCL2 and Cancer

Apoptosis, or programed cell death, is a stereotypical process ubiquitous to all eukaryotic organisms [15]. Apoptosis culminates in the activation of proteolytic enzymes (caspases) that irreversibly commit the cell to death. Failure of this process is a recognized hallmark of malignancy [16, 17] which drives not only the development of malignancy but also resistance to chemotherapy and radiotherapy [18–23].

There are two major pathways of apoptotic cell death: (1) the extrinsic pathway in which intracellular signaling cascades, that culminate in caspase activation, are triggered by extracellular death signals [24] and; (2) the intrinsic pathway which is the pathway most commonly perturbed in B cell malignancy.

Central to the intrinsic pathway of apoptosis is the BCL2 (B cell lymphoma 2) family of intra-cellular proteins that are characterized by conserved sequences in up to four BCL2 homology (BH) domains. This family is divided into three subgroups: pro-apoptotic BH3-only proteins; pro-survival proteins like BCL2; and apoptotic mediators. These three sub-groups interact specifically with one and other to trigger cell death (Fig. 1). In essence, it is the balance between the pro-survival and pro-apoptotic members of the BCL2 family that ultimately determines cellular fate [25].

The pro-apoptotic BH3-only proteins are activated by cellular stress signals including cytokine deprivation, oxidative stress, DNA-damage from chemotherapy or radiation, and proliferative stress. These proteins include BIM, BID, PUMA, and NOXA. When activated they bind selectively to [25] and inhibit the pro-survival BCL2 proteins. Under some circumstances they can also interact directly with the pro-apoptotic mediators to promote cell death.

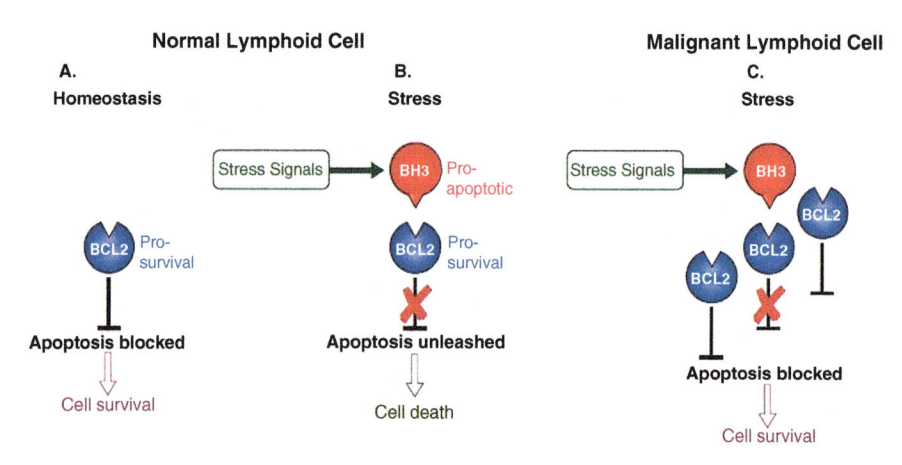

Fig. 1 In a normal healthy lymphoid cell the BCL2 pro-survival family of proteins block apoptosis and keep the cell alive (**a**) Under conditions of stress the BH3 only pro-apoptotic family of proteins are activated thus inhibiting the BCL2 family and unleashing apoptosis and cell death (**b**) In a malignant lymphoid cell however, BCL2 overexpression can overwhelm the capacity of the BH3 only proteins to trigger cell death resulting in inappropriate cell survival (**c**) *Figure created for Anderson, Seminars in Haematology, 2014* [24] (*Adapted from Chen et al. 2005* [25])

Fig. 2 Binding of BH3 mimetics to the BCL2 family (*Figure adapted from Chen, Cell, 2005* [25])

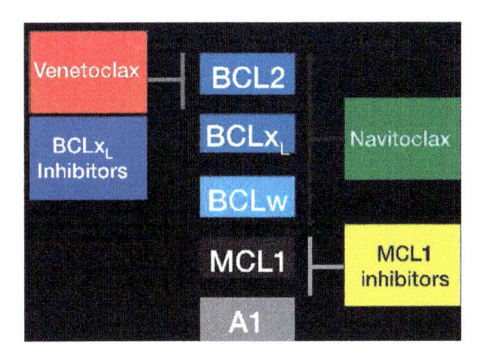

The pro-survival BCL2 proteins include: BCL2, BCLx$_L$, BCLw, MCL1 and A1. These proteins are bound by specific BH3-only family members. For instance, BAD binds to BCL2, BCLx$_L$ and BCLw, while NOXA binds to MCL1 and A1 and BIM binds to all BCL2 family members [25]. This selective BCL2 binding to the BH3-only proteins can now be therapeutically mimicked (Fig. 2). The BCL2 family acts to prevent cell death by binding to and inhibiting the pro-apoptotic mediators. The family members of this group are differentially expressed in various tissues throughout the body, and act to maintain tissue-specific cell survival. For instance, BCL2 is critical for the survival of lymphocytes at various stages in their development [26, 27], whereas BCLx$_L$ is critical to the survival of circulating platelets [28], and MCL1 is essential for plasma cell survival [29].

The final group of proteins that comprises the BCL2 family are the apoptotic mediators, which comprise the proteins BAK and BAX. These proteins are activated by removal of the BCL2 brake on their function. When active BAK and BAX trigger the mitochondrial outer membrane permeabilization is induced with cytochrome C release. Cytochrome C is an essential co-factor for caspase activation. The absence of BAK and BAX renders a cell resistant to apoptotic cell death via the intrinsic pathway [30, 31].

A direct consequence of BCL2 overexpression within a cell is quenching of the capacity of the BH3-only proteins to trigger apoptosis. Mechanistically, this underpins the inappropriate survival of cells in which BCL2 is overexpressed, and helps to explain why BCL2 overexpression can be such a powerful contributor both to malignancy and chemotherapy resistance. The role of BCL2 overexpression in malignancy was first elucidated in follicular lymphoma (FL) where the near universal presence of t(14;18), translocating the *IGVH* promoter to the *BCL2* gene, results in constitutive BCL2 overexpression [32, 33]. CLL has a high level of BCL2 expression [34], driven by the loss of mir15/16 mRNAs [35]. In CLL, the accumulation of BCL2 is thought to be central to the accumulation of malignant cells. While the critical role of BCL2 overexpression in driving resistance to apoptosis is best recognized in CLL and FL, BCL2 is commonly highly expressed in multiple B cell malignancies including multiple myeloma (MM) [36], mantle cell lymphoma (MCL) [37], Waldenstrom's macroglobulinemia (WM) [38] and diffuse large B cell lymphoma (DLBCL) [39].

BH3 Mimetics

Targeting BCL2 for the treatment of B cell malignancies has long been a goal of researchers as a way of enhancing the outcomes of chemotherapy among this group of patients. A true BH3 mimetic has been defined by Lessene et al. [40] as a drug that meets four key criteria: (*i*) apoptosis is via BAK/BAX with mitochrondrial disruption; (*ii*) the drug binds at least one BCL2 protein with high affinity; (*iii*) the drugs' activity correlates with its expression of relevant BCL2 family members and; (*iv*) relevant biomarkers are affected by the drug in animal models. The advent of nuclear magnetic resonance technology [41] greatly enhanced the structural understanding of the binding between the BH3-only proteins and the BCL2 family, this facilitated the development of the first true BH3 mimetic agent – ABT-737.

ABT-737

First described in 2005, ABT-737 is a small molecule prototype analogue for the BH3-only protein BAD [42] (Table 1). Like the physiologic intracellular protein BAD, ABT-737 binds to BCL2, BCLx$_L$ and BCLw with high affinity (Ki < 1 nM), with much lower binding affinity for MCL1 (Ki > 500 nM) [42]. The in vitro cytotoxicity of ABT-737 is dependent upon BAX and BAK [48], the sensitivity of malignant cells to the drug the correlates with expression of BCL2, BCLx$_L$ and BCLw [49] and it achieves both in vivo and in vitro efficacies against a range of B cell malignancies [42, 49–52]. However, ABT-737 was not suitable for oral administration due to solubility issues, and did not enter clinical trials.

Navitoclax

Navitoclax (also known as ABT-263) is an orally available analogue of ABT-737 [43] that entered clinical trials in 2007. Like ABT-737, navitoclax binds with high affinity to BCL2, BCLx$_L$ and BCLw (Ki < 1 nM) with minimal binding to MCL1 and A1 [43] and has pre-clinical evidence of efficacy against B cell malignancies [53].

The first-in-human trial of navitoclax amongst patients with relapsed/refractory B cell malignancies (including DLBCL, MCL, FL, CLL, peripheral NK/T cell lymphoma and Hodgkin lymphoma [HL]) demonstrated an overall response rate (ORR) of 22% (all partial responses [PRs]) with a median progression free survival (PFS) of 16 months [44]. However, there were few objective responses in diseases other than CLL/small lymphocytic lymphoma (SLL). When navitoclax was tested exclusively in patients with relapsed/refractory CLL/SLL it was associated with a 35% ORR (all PR) and a median PFS of 25 months [45].

Table 1 Comparison of BH3 mimetics

		ABT-737 nM [42]	Navitoclax nM [43–45]	Venetoclax nM [46, 47]
Target Binding (Ki)	BCL2	<1	<1	<0.0
	BCLx$_L$	<1	<1	48
	MCL1	460	>500	>444
CLL Clinical Efficacy	ORR	Did not enter clinical trials	35%	79%
	PR		35%	59%
	CR/CRi		0%	20%
	Median PFS		25 months	Median not reached; 69% (15 months)
NHL Clinical Efficacy	ORR	NA	22%	44%[a]
	PR		22%	13%
	CR/CRi		0%	31%
	Median PFS		16 months	Varied according to subtype[b]
CLL G3/G4 Haem AEs	Neutropenia	NA	28%	41%
	Thrombocytopenia		18% (G4)	12%
	Anemia			12%
NHL G3/G4 Haem AEs	Neutropenia	NA	18%	11%
	Thrombocytopenia		29%	<15%
	Lymphopenia		14%	<15%
	Anemia			15%
Dose Limiting Toxicity (DLT)		NA	Thrombocytopenia	In CLL tumor lysis syndrome, tolerated with ramp up dose scheduling In NHL: no DLT identified In MM: no DLT identified

Table adapted from Anderson, Seminars in Haematology, 2014 [24]. *nM* nano molar, *ORR* Overall response rate, *PR* Partial response, *CR* Complete response, *CRi* Complete response with incomplete marrow recovery, *PFS* Progression free survival, *NA* not applicable, *G3* Grade 3, *G4* Grade 4 *AE* Adverse event, *CLL* Chronic lymphocytic leukemia, *NHL* Non-Hodgkin lymphoma, *MM* multiple myeloma
[a]Response rates varied with disease subtype: mantel cell lymphoma ORR 44%, CR 13%; follicular lymphoma ORR 38%, CR 14%; diffuse large B cell lymphoma ORR 18%, CR 12%
[b]The estimated PFS for all patients was 6 months by subtype it was: 14 months for mantle cell lymphoma; 11 months for follicular lymphoma; and 1 month for diffuse large B cell lymphoma

While these results were promising even better outcomes were achieved when navitoclax was used as combination therapy. When used in combination with rituximab in CD20[+] lymphoproliferative disorders there was a 75% ORR with 5 out of 12 patients achieving a complete response (CR) [54]. In a randomized trial of navitoclax plus rituximab versus rituximab alone for previously untreated CLL, unsuitable for cytotoxic therapy, single agent rituximab achieved a 35% ORR in comparison to the combination arm where there was a 70% ORR (p = 0.03) [55]. Similarly, enhanced results were achieved when navitoclax was used in combination with bendamustine and rituximab in patients with relapsed/refractory CLL with 35% CR rate and 44% PR rate [56].

In a subset of patients treated on the phase I trial of navitoclax as a single agent in CLL, BCL2 family members were measured at baseline using western blotting [45]. In keeping with the literature, BCL2 was highly expressed at baseline in most samples, whereas MCL1 was expressed only in some samples. Importantly, however, there was no correlation between the objective clinical response and the expression of MCL1 or BCL2 at baseline [45]. However higher MCL1 levels did predict for a lesser reduction in lymphocytosis and high BIM:MCL1 ratios were associated with patients achieving an objective clinical response (all PRs) [45]. However, it was evident from very early in its clinical development that navitoclax was consistently associated with dose-proportional reductions in platelet counts and that thrombocytopenia was dose-limiting [44, 45]. Associated translational research demonstrated that $BCLx_L$ is critical for the survival of platelets in the peripheral circulation [28, 57], and that inhibition of BCLxL by navitoclax caused the thrombocytopenia. Thrombocytopenia precluded dose escalation of navitoclax above 300 mg daily, thus prohibiting the exploration of whether incremental improvements in clinical outcome could be achieved with higher doses.

Nevertheless, the promising clinical and preclinical data suggesting that inhibition of the BCL2 family was an effective therapeutic measure led to work to develop a BCL2 selective inhibitor. Unencumbered by $BCLx_L$-mediated thrombocytopenia, a BCL2 selective inhibitor was anticipated to allow greater dose escalation and more potent BCL2 inhibition with a safer hematological toxicity profile.

Venetoclax

Biochemistry

Venetoclax (also known as ABT-199) was developed by reverse engineering navitoclax to produce a compound which binds with high avidity to BCL2 (Ki <0.01 nM) but has much less avidity for $BCLx_L$ (Ki 43 nM) and BCLw (Ki 245 nM) with no measurable binding to MCL1 (Ki >444 nM) [46]. Venetoclax meets all the Lessene criteria for a true BH3 mimetic. It has no effect on double knock out BAX/BAK negative mouse embryonic fibroblasts [46], and kills normal and malignant B cells in a BAX/BAK-dependent fashion [58, 59]. Venetoclax demonstrates effective killing in the BCL2-dependent RS4;11 cell line, but not in the $BCLx_L$-dependent H146 cell line [46]. In cell lines, the cytotoxic effect of venetoclax is accompanied by markers of apoptotic cell death including cytochrome C release, activation of caspase 3/7 and phosphatidylserine exposure which was blocked by a pan-caspase inhibitor [46, 60]. Furthermore, venetoclax mediated killing is associated with disrupted BCL2-Bim, but not $BCLx_L$-Bim, complexes [46]. Cell death due to venetoclax was also proportional to the BCL2 expression [46].

Pre-clinical Data

Venetoclax killed CLL cells ex vivo at least as effectively as navitoclax, however ex vivo platelets were much less sensitive to death from venetoclax than navitoclax [46, 60] (Table 2). This translated to less in vivo platelet toxicity in dogs when treated with venetoclax compared to those treated with navitoclax [46]. Furthermore, killing of CLL cells by venetoclax has been shown to be via induction of apoptosis both in vitro and in vivo in patients. Venetoclax-mediated cytotoxicity is independent of the TP53 pathway function [61].

Table 2 Preclinical efficacy data

Disease model	*In vitro*	*In vivo*
Chronic lymphocytic leukemia	Primary CLL cells LC_{50}[a] 1.9 nM [61]	No accepted CLL cell line or appropriate murine model
Mantle cell lymphoma	3/8 MCL cell lines LD_{50}[b] <200 nM 10 primary MCL samples LD_{50} <10 nM [62]	In granta-519 xenografts tumor growth is inhibited by venetoclax [46]
Waldenstroms macroglobulinemia	CXCR4 mutations make WM resistant to ibrutinib In CXCR4 mutated WM cells sensitivity to ibrutinib enhanced by venetoclax [63]	
Follicular lymphoma	5 cell lines EC50 0.05 – 11 μM [46]	Toledo xenografts which harbor t(14:18) showed decreased tumor growth [46]
Diffuse large B cell lymphoma	20 cell lines EC_{50} 0.003 – 34.3 μM [46]	
Multiple myeloma	Primary myeloma cells harboring t(11;14) particularly sensitive [64]	
Acute lymphoblastic leukemia	4 cell lines EC_{50} 0.008 – 9.2 μM [46] Most ALL requires some $BCLx_L$ inhibition, however in MLL ALL venetoclax alone sufficient to induce cell killing [65]	In RS4;11 xenograft tumor growth inhibition and tumor delay dose dependent [46] *In vivo* MLL-ALL xenografts responded to venetoclax [65, 66]
Acute myeloid leukemia	In 2 cell lines EC_{50} 0.16 – 0.76 μM [46] Primary AML samples sensitive with median IC_{50}[c] 10 nmol/L, with death occurring within 2 h [67] Primary cells with IDH1 and IDH2 mutations were more sensitive compared with wild type [68]	Murine xenografts were sensitive [67]

Summary of pre-clinical venetoclax results in a variety of hematological malignancies
[a]50% lethality concentration
[b]50% lethal dose
[c]50% inhibitory concentration
MLL Mixed lineage leukemia

The near uniform overexpression of BCL2 in FL conferred by the presence of t(14;18) made this disease an obvious target for venetoclax. However, FL cell lines show variable sensitivity to venetoclax with half maximal effective concentrations (EC_{50}) ranging from 0.05–11 µM [46]. FL xenografts showed decreased tumor growth with venetoclax [46]. The more variable BCL2 expression in DLBCL is reflected in the fact that the sensitivity of DLBCL cell lines to venetoclax is highly variable with EC_{50}'s among 20 different cell lines ranging from 0.003 to 34.3 µM [46].

In MCL, 3 out of 8 cell lines were sensitive to venetoclax although intriguingly all primary samples tested showed sensitivity to this agent, possibly due to the fact that the primary samples were detached from the stroma with its protective niche [62]. WM cells with CXCR4 mutations are relatively resistant to ibrutinib. However, WM cells with CXCR4 mutations showed increased cell death when exposed to either ibrutinib or idealisib in combination with venetoclax [63]. Primary myeloma cells harboring t(11:14) appear uniformly sensitive to venetoclax [64].

ALL cell lines showed variable sensitivity to venetoclax with EC_{50}s ranging from 0.008 to 9.2 µM and in the RS4;11 xenograft model there was dose-dependent reduction in tumor growth in response to venetoclax [46]. Mixed lineage leukemia (MLL) ALL was sensitive to venetoclax alone [65, 66] raising the possibility of tailoring BCL2 inhibition to the individual leukemia subtype. Among AML cell lines the sensitivity to venetoclax ranged from EC_{50} 0.16 to 0.76 µM [46]. Primary AML samples died promptly and at low concentrations in response to venetoclax [67], especially AML cells with IDH1 (isocitrate dehydrogenase) and IDH2 mutations [68]. Similarly, AML xenografts were sensitive to venetoclax [67].

Administration and Pharmacokinetics

The phase I first-in-human study of venetoclax was a dose-finding study and tested oral venetoclax in CLL and NHL patients at once daily doses ranging between 150 and 1200 mg [47, 69]. The major toxicity associated with venetoclax in CLL was tumor lysis syndrome (TLS), which could be ameliorated by the implementation of slow dose escalation along with routine xanthine oxidase inhibition and hydration [47]. No maximum tolerated dose (MTD) was identified. In CLL, the recommended phase II dose (RP2D) was 400 mg daily [47].

The peak plasma concentrations of venetoclax were found at 6–8 h post first dose and the half-life after a single 50 mg dose was 19 h [47]. The steady state exposure to venetoclax is proportional to dose. Importantly, the pharmacokinetics of venetoclax were not affected by co-administration with rituximab [70].

Clinical Outcomes

In the phase I first-in-human study of venetoclax among 116 patients with relapsed/refractory CLL or SLL treated with venetoclax monotherapy [47] the ORR across all risk subgroups was 79% despite being a study heavily enriched for poor prognosis

CLL [47] with a 20% CR rate and 5% of patients who achieved bone marrow minimal residual disease (MRD) negativity by flow cytometry. While these results are very encouraging the reported cumulative rate of disease progression after a median of 17 months was 35%, with 16% of patients experiencing a Richter's transformation (RT) (most commonly to DLBCL) [47]. The 2 year overall survival (OS) estimate was 84% and the 15 months PFS estimate at a dose of 400 mg daily was 69%, with a median PFS of 25 months (95% confidence interval [CI] 17–30 months) among the dose escalation cohort [47]. Despite equivalent overall response rates, progression appeared to be more common among patients with del17p. In patients with del17p the median PFS was only 16 months (95% CI 11–25 months) in contrast to those without del17p among whom the median PFS was not reached (estimated at 71% at 15 months) [47]. The duration of response was longer among those who achieved a CR compared with those whose best response was PR [47].

These findings were confirmed in a phase II open label study of venetoclax among relapsed/refractory CLL patients with del17p in which 107 patients were treated with 400 mg orally once a day [71]. There was a similar ORR and PFS amongst all prognostic categories with the response being unaffected by: refractoriness to prior therapies, proportion of cells with del17p, presence of *TP53* mutation and other poor prognostic markers [71]. Among all patients the median time on treatment was 12.1 months during which time 37 patients discontinued study drug. The reasons for discontinuation were disease progression in 24 (11 due to RT), adverse events in 9, withdrawal of consent in 2, non-compliance in 1 and allograft in three [71]. The estimated 12-month PFS was 72% with an estimated 12-month OS of 86.7%, an estimated 12-month event free survival (EFS) of 70% and a 12-month time to progression (TTP) of 77% [71]. Among the patients achieving CR, 100% continued to respond to venetoclax at 12 months on study. Among the 24 patients with progressive disease the TTP was shorter in the patients who progressed with RT (4.7 months) compared to the patients who progressed with CLL (6.3 months) [71]. Interestingly in a sub-group analysis of patients who had previously progressed on ibrutinib or idealisib, the majority of these patients responded to venetoclax [71].

Venetoclax (200–600 mg) has also been tested in combination with rituximab (monthly for 6 months) in a phase Ib dose finding study of 49 patients with relapsed/refractory CLL [70]. In this study, the ORR was 86% with improved rates of CR (51%) of whom 80% of patients were negative on MRD testing [70]. As with the single agent studies similar OR and CR rates were seen across all prognostic groups analyzed. In this study, disease progression on treatment was seen in 11/49 patients. Among these 6 progressed with CLL (all patients in whom the best response was PR) and 5 progressed with RT (all transformations were seen at less than 9 months on study) [70]. However, the deeper responses seen with combination therapy and were associated with more enduring disease control; for instance, the 2 year estimates for freedom from progression (FFP) and ongoing response were 82% and 89%, respectively [70]. The TTP was not reached in this study but the 2-year progression free estimate was 82% (95% CI

66–91 months). The two-year estimate for ongoing response was 89% (95% CI 72–96 months) with deeper responses being more durable [70]. For instance, the 2-year estimate for ongoing CR was 100% (95% CI 100–100) while those for ongoing PR or MRD positive disease response were 73% (95% CI 42–89) or 71% (95% CI 39–88), respectively.

Deep and enduring responses raise the possibility of prolonged remissions or even 'cure' with combination therapy. Hence, 13 CLL patients on the phase Ib study of venetoclax in combination with rituximab who achieved either CR or PR with bone marrow MRD negativity discontinued venetoclax. At the time of publication 11 patients who were MRD negative remained off treatment with no evidence of progression. The two patients who were MRD positive developed disease progression after 24 months off treatment but then responded to re-institution of therapy with venetoclax [70].

The phase I first-in-human study of venetoclax monotherapy also included an arm for 106 patients with relapsed/refractory NHL treated in dose escalation and safety expansion cohorts at doses from 200 to 1200 mg daily [69]. The study encompassed a diverse range of lymphomas including MCL, FL, DLBCL, DLBCL due to RT, WM and marginal zone lymphoma (MZL). The ORR for the study was 44%. However, the response rates varied with the NHL subtype, for instance: MCL ORR was 75% with 21% CR; FL ORR was 38% with 14% CR; DLBCL ORR was 18% with 12% CR; in RT DLBCL ORR was 43% with no CR; MZL ORR was 67% with no CR; and WM ORR was 100% with no CR [69].

In keeping with the CLL findings, among patients achieving CR the responses appeared more durable than those in patients whose best response was PR. Also in keeping with the findings from navitoclax testing in CLL, the strength of BCL2 expression by immunohistochemistry (IHC) did not correlate with resistance to venetoclax among NHL patients [69].

At the time of publication 87/106 NHL patients had discontinued the study due to: progressive disease (PD) (77), adverse events (3), change in management to allograft (3), withdrawal of consent (2) and non-compliance/investigator decision (2) [69]. Among these, 87 patients exiting study, 38 have subsequently died; 10 within 30 days of coming off study (all due to PD) and 28 at more than 30 days after coming off study (among whom 24 died of PD) [69].

In a phase I study of venetoclax in combination with the proteasome inhibitor bortezomib, which can indirectly inhibit MCL [72, 73], an ORR of 50% with a median DOR of 5–9 months (range 0–14.1 months) was observed among 41 patients with relapsed/refractory myeloma. Efficacy was largely restricted to patients who were either bortezomib naive or had responded to previous exposure to bortezomib [74].

In a phase Ib study of venetoclax in combination with decitabine or azacitidine in treatment naive elderly patients with AML, among 19 evaluable patients there were 14 CRs, 2 PRs and 3 resistant. During the follow-up period no relapses were seen among the patients who achieved objective responses [75].

Clinical Effect of Resistance

Our group has recently analyzed 67 treated patients with venetoclax for relapsed/refractory CLL/SLL [76]. Twenty-five (37%) patients progressed during a median follow up of 23 months of whom 17 had a RT; 14 DLBCL and 3 HL [76]. RT was manifested by B symptoms with or without cytopenias in 3 cases and by asymptomatic progressive lymphadenopathy in 14 cases [76]. In the majority of patients with RT PET scans revealed multifocal sites of FDG avidity and in all cases of DLBLC RT BCL2 overexpression was present on immunohistochemistry [76]. The median time to progression with RT was 7.9 months compared with 23.4 months for those who progressed with CLL (p = 0.003) [76]. On univariate analysis the highest risk for progression was seen among patients with either fludarabine refractory disease or complex cytogenetics [76]. Other high risk features such as advanced age, multiple lines of prior therapy, deletion 17p, deletion 11q and TP53 mutations were not associated with the risk of progression [76].

Six of 8 patients with progressive CLL/SLL on venetoclax were subsequently treated with ibrutinib and of these five achieved a PR with three remaining alive on therapy at 6, 6, and 9 months of follow up [76]. The treatments for RT included chemotherapy followed by consolidation with autograph (2), allograft (2) or radiotherapy (2) [76]. A further 10 patients with RT received chemotherapy alone and one patient was managed with palliative care alone [76]. Three patients with DLBCL RT who responded to salvage therapy subsequently progressed with CLL/SLL and remain alive on BTK inhibitors at 30, 34, and 38 months [76]. Median post progression survival for HL RT, DLBCL RT and progressive CLL/SLL was not reached, 10.9 and 8.6 months respectively [76].

In the phase I first in human study of venetoclax in relapsed/refractory NHL the estimated PFS for 106 patients was 6 months (95% CI 4–10 months). However, PFS varied by histology being longer in disease subtypes associated with deeper clinical responses; for example, the median PFSs were 14, 11, and 1 months for MCL, FL and DLBCL, respectively [69]. In WM, the DOR varied from 11.1–41.5 months and in MZL it varied from 2.3–23.6 months. Overall, the estimated 12 month OS was 70% but varied by subtype being 100%, 82% and 32% for FL, MCL and DLBCL, respectively [77].

Molecular Mechanisms of Resistance

In CLL, in vivo mechanisms of resistance to BCL2 inhibitors are not yet fully elucidated but there are emerging clinical data pertaining to a heterogeneous group of implicated molecular pathways (Table 3). Identifying the molecular drivers of resistance is an area of active genomic research. While point mutations in the drug-binding site of the target protein BTK are a common form of resistance to the drug ibrutinib, to date analogous mutations in the drug-binding interface of BCL2 have not been identified in patients treated with venetoclax.

Table 3 Potential mechanisms of resistance to BCL2 inhibiting BH3 mimetics

	Cell lines	Mouse models	Primary samples
BCL2 mutations	Mouse lymphoma cells with BCL2 mutations resistant to venetoclax [78]		
BAX mutations	Mouse lymphoma cells with BAX mutations resistant to venetoclax [78]		
Reduced BCL2 expression	Resistant FL cell lines down regulate BCL2 [79]		
Up-regulation MCL1 + BCLx$_L$ expression	MCL1 and BCLx$_L$ conferred resistance to venetoclax in MCL cells cultured on fibroblasts this was lost when cells were detached from fibroblasts [62] In myeloma cell lines resistance is mediated by MCL1 and sensitivity is correlated with high BCL2, low BCLx$_L$ and low MCL1 [80] In human tumor cell lines cyclin E depletion with CDK inhibitors decreased MCL1 protein levels restoring sensitivity to BH3 mimetics [81]	Multiple myeloma xenografts that co-expressed BCLx$_L$ or MCL1 with BCL2 were resistant to venetoclax [80] In a variety of ALL xenograft models there was increased killing with dual BCLx$_L$ and BCL2 inhibition compared with BCL2 inhibition with venetoclax alone [65]	MCL cells mobilized in patients treated with ibrutinib were highly sensitive to venetoclax [62] In primary CLL cells BCR signaling up-regulates MCL1 conferring resistance to venetoclax. This can be overcome by SYK inhibitors which prevent BCR mediated MCL1 induction [82]
Micro-environment mediated protection			CLL cultured on a stromal growth layer is resistant to venetoclax, this is overcome by co administration of anti CD20 antibodies [83] When MCL cells were cultured in a lymphoid like environment they become resistant to venetoclax; this can be overcome with co-treatment using the anti CD20 antibody obinutuzumab [84]

(continued)

Table 3 (continued)

	Cell lines	Mouse models	Primary samples
ERK activation	In FL cell lines activation of ERK protects against venetoclax induced apoptosis inhibition of PI3κ increased apoptosis due to venetoclax [79]		

Summary of representative published data for purported mechanisms of resistance to BH3 mimetics

In BCL2 mutations render mouse lymphoma cells resistant to venetoclax [78]. Acquired mutations in BCL2 family proteins have also been shown to confer in vitro resistance to venetoclax in lymphoma cell lines [78]. However, we have looked specifically for these mutations among our resistant CLL patients and to date we have been unable to demonstrate an association between mutations in BCL2 and venetoclax resistance (unpublished).

Previous studies utilizing IHC [69] and protein expression by western blotting [45] have failed to demonstrate a strong correlation between resistance to BH3 mimetics in patients and the protein expression of family members within the malignant cells. To date only preliminary ad hoc analysis of IHC is available at the time of CLL progression on venetoclax. In work by our group, (unpublished), all 14 patients with DLBCL RT were IHC positive for BCL2. This suggests that, at least in DLBCL RT, BCL2 down regulation is not the mechanism underlying disease progression.

Among NHL patients in the phase I study, 41/46 patients assessed had high BCL2 expression by IHC and this was not correlated with either best response or PFS [69]. High BCL2 IHC expression was seen in all NHL subtypes including MCL, FL, DLBCL and WM (all >75%) [69]. When both BCL2 and c-MYC expression were assessed by IHC among the DLBCL patients, the double expresser status did not predict for an objective response either [69].

Increased MCL1 and $BCLx_L$ expressions have been associated with resistance of MCL cells to venetoclax when cultured on fibroblasts; this resistance, however, is lost if the cells are detached [62]. Similarly, MCL cells mobilized in vivo by ibrutinib are sensitive to venetoclax [62]. In myeloma cell lines, MCL1 can mediate resistance to venetoclax and targeting MCL1 results in the death of 70% of myeloma cells [59]. In primary myeloma cells, sensitivity to venetoclax is correlated with increased BCL2, reduced $BCLx_L$ and reduced MCL1 [80]. Reducing MCL1 with CDK inhibitors can overcome resistance to BH3 mimetics in human tumor cells [81]. MCL1 expression may account for the relatively poor response of non t(11;14) multiple myeloma to venetoclax monotherapy [85] compared with the higher response rates seen when it is combined with bortezomib [74], which can down regulate MCL1. In vitro, increased MCL1 from B cell receptor signaling (BCR) in

CLL results in venetoclax resistance, which can be overcome by SYK inhibition, (which deceases BCR mediated MCL1 induction) [82].

In non MLL ALL, venetoclax alone resulted in fewer objective responses among xenografts compared to dual $BCLx_L$ and BCL2 inhibition [65]. Resistant FL cell lines have been associated with reduced BCL2 [79]. BAX mutations in mouse lymphoma can also result in resistance to venetoclax [78]. Among AML patients receiving venetoclax monotherapy BH3 profiling was able to predict for patients likely to be more sensitive to venetoclax, however, it did not predict for longer duration of resistance [86]. In this study, the best predictor of sustained response was reduced $BCLx_L$ and MCL1 functions [86]. BH3 profiling using Bim peptide as a measure of mitochondrial priming for apoptosis suggested that patients with increased mitochondrial priming had better in vivo responses to venetoclax [61] and this technique may emerge as a way of predicting for venetoclax resistance. However, protein expression studies have so far been unable to demonstrate an association between relative expression of MCL1, BCL2 or $BCLx_L$ and clinical outcomes in either CLL or NHL patients treated with BH3 mimetics [45, 69].

The microenvironment can also confer resistance to venetoclax and this appears to be overcome by anti CD20 antibodies in both CLL [83] and MCL [84]. In FL xenografts the acquired resistance to venetoclax can be overcome by the addition of rituximab [79]. Furthermore, in FL cell lines the activation of ERK protects from venetoclax-induced apoptosis and this can be overcome by PI3κ inhibitors [79]. Collectively, this suggests that at least some forms of resistance to venetoclax may be overcome by rational drug combinations.

Conclusion

Venetoclax represents a significant step forward in the management of high-risk CLL and potentially a number of other hematological malignancies. However, a percentage of patients continue to be primary refractory to this agent and even among responders the PFS can be limited. Understanding the mechanisms for clinical resistance will be critical to improving outcomes for patients. It is hoped that targeting multiple intracellular cancer pathways through rational drug combinations will improve both response rates and duration of response. Proof of this concept has already been shown in CLL with the combination of rituximab and venetoclax resulting in deeper and longer lasting responses compared to monotherapy with either agent alone [70]. Venetoclax combination studies are currently underway in a variety of disease subtypes and in a variety of combinations including: with ibrutinib in CLL and MCL (NCT02756897 and NCT02419560); with bortezomib in multiple myeloma [74]; and in combination with standard chemotherapy in NHL (NCT02055820). Identifying biomarkers for resistance will help to target which patients require combination therapies for optimal results.

Ongoing clinical trials are being undertaken to address all these questions. Enhanced molecular understanding of the genetic features of CLL determining depth of response to venetoclax, and progression of disease while on treatment with this agent, will be necessary to identify which patients are most likely to benefit and to target combinations to optimize long-term outcome.

Conflict of Interests MAA and AWR are employees of the Walter and Eliza Hall Institute of Medical Research which receives milestone and royalty payments related to venetoclax.

References

1. Coiffier B, Lepage E, Briere J, et al. CHOP chemotherapy plus rituximab compared with CHOP alone in elderly patients with diffuse large-B-cell lymphoma. N Engl J Med. 2002;346:235–42.
2. Byrd JC, Rai K, Peterson BL, et al. Addition of rituximab to fludarabine may prolong progression-free survival and overall survival in patients with previously untreated chronic lymphocytic leukemia: an updated retrospective comparative analysis of CALGB 9712 and CALGB 9011. Blood. 2005;105:49–53.
3. Döhner H, Stilgenbauer S, Benner A, et al. Genomic aberrations and survival in chronic lymphocytic leukemia. N Engl J Med. 2000;343:1910–6.
4. Mayr C, Speicher MR, Kofler DM, et al. Chromosomal translocations are associated with poor prognosis in chronic lymphocytic leukemia. Blood. 2006;107:742–51.
5. Tam CS, O'Brien S, Lerner S, et al. The natural history of fludarabine-refractory chronic lymphocytic leukemia patients who fail alemtuzumab or have bulky lymphadenopathy. Leuk Lymphoma. 2007;48:1931–9.
6. Zenz T, Gribben JG, Hallek M, et al. Risk categories and refractory CLL in the era of chemoimmunotherapy. Blood. 2012;119:4101–7.
7. Robak T, Dmoszynska A, Solal-Celigny P, et al. Rituximab plus fludarabine and cyclophosphamide prolongs progression-free survival compared with fludarabine and cyclophosphamide alone in previously treated chronic lymphocytic leukemia. J Clin Oncol. 2010;28:1756–65.
8. Keating MJ, O'Brien S, Kantarjian H, et al. Long-term follow-up of patients with chronic lymphocytic leukemia treated with fludarabine as a single agent. Blood. 1993;81:2878–84.
9. Tam CS, O'Brien S, Wierda W, et al. Long-term results of the fludarabine, cyclophosphamide, and rituximab regimen as initial therapy of chronic lymphocytic leukemia. Blood. 2008;112:975–80.
10. Hamblin TJ, Davis Z, Gardiner A, et al. Unmutated Ig V(H) genes are associated with a more aggressive form of chronic lymphocytic leukemia. Blood. 1999;94:1848–54.
11. Byrd JC, Furman RR, Coutre SE, et al. Targeting BTK with ibrutinib in relapsed chronic lymphocytic leukemia. N Engl J Med. 2013;369:32–42.
12. Brown JR, Byrd JC, Coutre SE, et al. Idelalisib, an inhibitor of phosphatidylinositol 3-kinase p110delta, for relapsed/refractory chronic lymphocytic leukemia. Blood. 2014;123:3390–7.
13. Gopal AK, Kahl BS, de Vos S, et al. PI3Kdelta inhibition by idelalisib in patients with relapsed indolent lymphoma. N Engl J Med. 2014;370:1008–18.
14. Burger JA, Tedeschi A, Barr PM, et al. Ibrutinib as initial therapy for patients with chronic lymphocytic leukemia. N Engl J Med. 2015;373:2425–37.
15. Hotchkiss RS, Strasser A, McDunn JE, Swanson PE. Cell death. N Engl J Med. 2009;361:1570–83.
16. Hanahan D, Weinberg RA. The hallmarks of cancer. Cell. 2000;100:57–70.
17. Hanahan D, Weinberg RA. Hallmarks of cancer: the next generation. Cell. 2011;144:646–74.
18. Strasser A, Harris AW, Jacks T, Cory S. DNA damage can induce apoptosis in proliferating lymphoid cells via p53-independent mechanisms inhibitable by Bcl-2. Cell. 1994;79:329–39.

19. Schmitt CA, Rosenthal CT, Lowe SW. Genetic analysis of chemoresistance in primary murine lymphomas. Nat Med. 2000;6:1029–35.
20. Huang DC, O'Reilly LA, Strasser A, Cory S. The anti-apoptosis function of Bcl-2 can be genetically separated from its inhibitory effect on cell cycle entry. EMBO J. 1997;16:4628–38.
21. Miyashita T, Reed JC. Bcl-2 gene transfer increases relative resistance of S49.1 and WEHI7.2 lymphoid cells to cell death and DNA fragmentation induced by glucocorticoids and multiple chemotherapeutic drugs. Cancer Res. 1992;52:5407–11.
22. Miyashita T, Reed JC. Bcl-2 oncoprotein blocks chemotherapy-induced apoptosis in a human leukemia cell line. Blood. 1993;81:151–7.
23. Kamesaki S, Kamesaki H, Jorgensen TJ, et al. Bcl-2 protein inhibits etoposide-induced apoptosis through its effects on events subsequent to topoisomerase II-induced DNA strand breaks and their repair. Cancer Res. 1993;53:4251–6.
24. Anderson MA, Huang D, Roberts A. Targeting BCL2 for the treatment of lymphoid malignancies. Semin Hematol. 2014;51:219–27.
25. Chen L, Willis SN, Wei A, et al. Differential targeting of prosurvival Bcl-2 proteins by their BH3-only ligands allows complementary apoptotic function. Mol Cell. 2005;17:393–403.
26. Veis DJ, Sorenson CM, Shutter JR, Korsmeyer SJ. Bcl-2-deficient mice demonstrate fulminant lymphoid apoptosis, polycystic kidneys, and hypopigmented hair. Cell. 1993;75:229–40.
27. Merino D, Khaw SL, Glaser SP, et al. Bcl-2, Bcl-x(L), and Bcl-w are not equivalent targets of ABT-737 and navitoclax (ABT-263) in lymphoid and leukemic cells. Blood. 2012;119:5807–16.
28. Mason KD, Carpinelli MR, Fletcher JI, et al. Programmed anuclear cell death delimits platelet life span. Cell. 2007;128:1173–86.
29. Peperzak V, Vikstrom I, Walker J, et al. Mcl-1 is essential for the survival of plasma cells. Nat Immunol. 2013;14:290–7.
30. Wei MC, Zong WX, Cheng EH, et al. Proapoptotic BAX and BAK: a requisite gateway to mitochondrial dysfunction and death. Science. 2001;292:727–30.
31. Zong WX, Lindsten T, Ross AJ, et al. BH3-only proteins that bind pro-survival Bcl-2 family members fail to induce apoptosis in the absence of Bax and Bak. Genes Dev. 2001;15:1481–6.
32. Tsujimoto Y, Cossman J, Jaffe E, Croce CM. Involvement of the bcl-2 gene in human follicular lymphoma. Science. 1985;228:1440–3.
33. Tsujimoto Y, Croce CM. Recent progress on the human bcl-2 gene involved in follicular lymphoma: characterization of the protein products. Curr Top Microbiol Immunol. 1988;141:337–40.
34. Robertson LE, Plunkett W, McConnell K, et al. Bcl-2 expression in chronic lymphocytic leukemia and its correlation with the induction of apoptosis and clinical outcome. Leukemia. 1996;10:456–9.
35. Calin GA, Dumitru CD, Shimizu M, et al. Frequent deletions and down-regulation of micro-RNA genes miR15 and miR16 at 13q14 in chronic lymphocytic leukemia. Proc Natl Acad Sci. 2002;99:15524–9.
36. Pettersson M, Jernberg-Wiklund H, Larsson LG, et al. Expression of the bcl-2 gene in human multiple myeloma cell lines and normal plasma cells. Blood. 1992;79:495–502.
37. Agarwal B, Naresh KN. Bcl-2 family of proteins in indolent B-cell non-Hodgkin's lymphoma: study of 116 cases. Am J Hematol. 2002;70:278–82.
38. Vijay A, Gertz MA. Waldenstrom macroglobulinemia. Blood. 2007;109:5096–103.
39. Aisenberg AC, Wilkes BM, Jacobson JO. The bcl-2 gene is rearranged in many diffuse B-cell lymphomas. Blood. 1988;71:969–72.
40. Lessene G, Czabotar PE, Colman PM. BCL-2 family antagonists for cancer therapy. Nat Rev Drug Discov. 2008;7:989–1000.
41. Shuker SB, Hajduk PJ, Meadows RP, Fesik SW. Discovering high-affinity ligands for proteins: SAR by NMR. Science. 1996;274:1531–4.
42. Oltersdorf T, Elmore SW, Shoemaker AR, et al. An inhibitor of Bcl-2 family proteins induces regression of solid tumours. Nature. 2005;435:677–81.

43. Tse C, Shoemaker AR, Adickes J, et al. ABT-263: a potent and orally bioavailable Bcl-2 family inhibitor. Cancer Res. 2008;68:3421–8.
44. Wilson WH, O'Connor OA, Czuczman MS, et al. Navitoclax, a targeted high-affinity inhibitor of BCL-2, in lymphoid malignancies: a phase 1 dose-escalation study of safety, pharmacokinetics, pharmacodynamics, and antitumour activity. Lancet Oncol. 2010;11:1149–59.
45. Roberts AW, Seymour JF, Brown JR, et al. Substantial susceptibility of chronic lymphocytic leukemia to BCL2 inhibition: results of a phase I study of navitoclax in patients with relapsed or refractory disease. J Clin Oncol. 2012;30:488–96.
46. Souers AJ, Leverson JD, Boghaert ER, et al. ABT-199, a potent and selective BCL-2 inhibitor, achieves antitumor activity while sparing platelets. Nat Med. 2013;19:202–8.
47. Roberts AW, Davids MS, Pagel JM, et al. Targeting BCL2 with Venetoclax in relapsed chronic lymphocytic leukemia. N Engl J Med. 2016;374:311–22.
48. van Delft MF, Wei AH, Mason KD, et al. The BH3 mimetic ABT-737 targets selective Bcl-2 proteins and efficiently induces apoptosis via Bak/Bax if Mcl-1 is neutralized. Cancer Cell. 2006;10:389–99.
49. Mason KD, Vandenberg CJ, Scott CL, et al. In vivo efficacy of the Bcl-2 antagonist ABT-737 against aggressive Myc-driven lymphomas. Proc Natl Acad Sci USA. 2008;105:17961–6.
50. Kang MH, Kang YH, Szymanska B, et al. Activity of vincristine, L-ASP, and dexamethasone against acute lymphoblastic leukemia is enhanced by the BH3-mimetic ABT-737 in vitro and in vivo. Blood. 2007;110:2057–66.
51. Kline MP, Rajkumar SV, Timm MM, et al. ABT-737, an inhibitor of Bcl-2 family proteins, is a potent inducer of apoptosis in multiple myeloma cells. Leukemia. 2007;21:1549–60.
52. Mason KD, Khaw SL, Rayeroux KC, et al. The BH3 mimetic compound, ABT-737, synergizes with a range of cytotoxic chemotherapy agents in chronic lymphocytic leukemia. Leukemia. 2009;23:2034–41.
53. Ackler S, Mitten MJ, Foster K, et al. The Bcl-2 inhibitor ABT-263 enhances the response of multiple chemotherapeutic regimens in hematologic tumors in vivo. Cancer Chemother Pharmacol. 2010;66:869–80.
54. Roberts AW, Advani RH, Kahl BS, et al. Phase 1 study of the safety, pharmacokinetics, and antitumour activity of the BCL2 inhibitor navitoclax in combination with rituximab in patients with relapsed or refractory CD20+ lymphoid malignancies. Br J Haematol. 2015;170:669–78.
55. Kipps TJ, Eradat H, Grosicki S, et al. A phase 2 study of the BH3 mimetic BCL2 inhibitor navitoclax (ABT-263) with or without rituximab, in previously untreated B-cell chronic lymphocytic leukemia. Leuk Lymphoma. 2015;56:2826–33.
56. Kipps TJ, Swinnen LJ, Wierda WG, et al. Navitoclax (ABT-263) plus Fludarabine/Cyclophosphamide/Rituximab (FCR) or Bendamustine/Rituximab (BR): a phase 1 study in patients with relapsed/refractory Chronic Lymphocytic Leukemia (CLL). Blood. 2011;118:3904.
57. Zhang H, Nimmer PM, Tahir SK, et al. Bcl-2 family proteins are essential for platelet survival. Cell Death Differ. 2007;14:943–51.
58. Khaw SL, Merino D, Anderson MA, et al. Both leukaemic and normal peripheral B lymphoid cells are highly sensitive to the selective pharmacological inhibition of prosurvival Bcl-2 with ABT-199. Leukemia. 2014;28:1207–15.
59. Gong JN, Khong T, Segal D, et al. Hierarchy for targeting pro-survival BCL2 family proteins in multiple myeloma: pivotal role of MCL1. Blood. 2016;14:1834–44.
60. Vogler M, Dinsdale D, Dyer MJ, Cohen GM. ABT-199 selectively inhibits BCL2 but not BCL2L1 and efficiently induces apoptosis of chronic lymphocytic leukaemic cells but not platelets. Br J Haematol. 2013;163:139–42.
61. Anderson MA, Deng J, Seymour JF, et al. The BCL2 selective inhibitor venetoclax induces rapid onset apoptosis of CLL cells in patients via a TP53 independent mechanism. Blood. 2016;127(25):3215–24.

62. Chiron D, Dousset C, Brosseau C, et al. Biological rational for sequential targeting of Bruton tyrosine kinase and Bcl-2 to overcome CD40-induced ABT-199 resistance in mantle cell lymphoma. Oncotarget. 2015;6:8750–9.
63. Cao Y, Hunter ZR, Liu X, et al. CXCR4 WHIM-like frameshift and nonsense mutations promote ibrutinib resistance but do not supplant MYD88(L265P) -directed survival signalling in Waldenstrom macroglobulinaemia cells. Br J Haematol. 2015;168:701–7.
64. Touzeau C, Dousset C, Le Gouill S, et al. The Bcl-2 specific BH3 mimetic ABT-199: a promising targeted therapy for t(11;14) multiple myeloma. Leukemia. 2014;28:210–2.
65. Khaw SL, Suryani S, Evans K, et al. Venetoclax responses of pediatric ALL xenografts reveal sensitivity of MLL-rearranged leukemia. Blood. 2016;128:1382–95.
66. Benito JM, Godfrey L, Kojima K, et al. MLL-rearranged acute lymphoblastic Leukemias activate BCL-2 through H3K79 methylation and are sensitive to the BCL-2-specific antagonist ABT-199. Cell Rep. 2015;13:2715–27.
67. Pan R, Hogdal LJ, Benito JM, et al. Selective BCL-2 inhibition by ABT-199 causes on-target cell death in acute myeloid leukemia. Cancer Discov. 2014;4:362–75.
68. Chan SM, Thomas D, Corces-Zimmerman MR, et al. Isocitrate dehydrogenase 1 and 2 mutations induce BCL-2 dependence in acute myeloid leukemia. Nat Med. 2015;21:178–84.
69. Davids M, Roberts A, Seymour J, et al. A phase I first-in-human study of venetoclax in patients with relapsed or refractory non-Hodgkin lymphoma. J Clin Oncol. 2017;35(8):826–33.
70. Seymour J, Ma S, Phase BD. 1b study of venetoclax plus rituximab in relapsed or refractory chronic lymphocytic leukaemia. Lancet Oncol. 2017;18(2):230–40.
71. Stilgenbauer S, Eichhorst B, Schetelig J, et al. Venetoclax in relapsed or refractory chronic lymphocytic leukaemia with 17p deletion: a multicentre, open-label, phase 2 study. Lancet Oncol. 2016;17(6):768–78.
72. Edwards SK, Han Y, Liu Y, et al. Signaling mechanisms of bortezomib in TRAF3-deficient mouse B lymphoma and human multiple myeloma cells. Leuk Res. 2016;41:85–95.
73. Qin JZ, Ziffra J, Stennett L, et al. Proteasome inhibitors trigger NOXA-mediated apoptosis in melanoma and myeloma cells. Cancer Res. 2005;65:6282–93.
74. Moreau P, Chanan-Khan A, Roberts AW, et al. Safety and efficacy of Venetoclax (ABT-199/GDC-0199) in combination with Bortezomib and dexamethasone in relapsed/refractory multiple myeloma: phase 1b results. Blood. 2015;126:3038–8.
75. DiNardo C, Pollyea D, Pratz K, et al. A phase 1b study of Venetoclax (ABT-199/GDC-0199) in combination with Decitabine or Azacitidine in treatment-naive patients with acute Myelogenous leukemia who are ≥ to 65 years and not eligible for standard induction therapy. Blood. 2015;126:327.
76. Lew TE, Anderson MA, Tam CS, et al. Clinicopathological features and outcomes of progression for Chronic Lymphocytic Leukaemia (CLL) treated with the BCL2 inhibitor venetoclax. Blood. 2016;128:3223.
77. Davids MS, Roberts AW, Seymour JF, et al. Safety, efficacy and immune effects of venetoclax 400 mg daily in patients with relapsed chronic lymphocytic leukemia (CLL). J Clin Oncol (Meeting Abstracts). 2016;34:7527.
78. Fresquet V, Rieger M, Carolis C, et al. Acquired mutations in BCL2 family proteins conferring resistance to the BH3 mimetic ABT-199 in lymphoma. Blood. 2014;123:4111–9.
79. Bodo J, Zhao X, Durkin L, et al. Acquired resistance to venetoclax (ABT-199) in t(14;18) positive lymphoma cells. Oncotarget. 2016;7:70000–10.
80. Punnoose EA, Leverson JD, Peale F, et al. Expression profile of BCL-2, BCL-XL, and MCL-1 predicts pharmacological response to the BCL-2 selective antagonist Venetoclax in multiple myeloma models. Mol Cancer Ther. 2016;15:1132–44.
81. Choudhary GS, Tat TT, Misra S, et al. Cyclin E/Cdk2-dependent phosphorylation of Mcl-1 determines its stability and cellular sensitivity to BH3 mimetics. Oncotarget. 2015;6:16912–25.
82. Bojarczuk K, Sasi BK, Gobessi S, et al. BCR signaling inhibitors differ in their ability to overcome Mcl-1-mediated resistance of CLL B cells to ABT-199. Blood. 2016;127:3192–201.

83. Thijssen R, Slinger E, Weller K, et al. Resistance to ABT-199 induced by microenvironmental signals in chronic lymphocytic leukemia can be counteracted by CD20 antibodies or kinase inhibitors. Haematologica. 2015;100:e302–6.
84. Chiron D, Bellanger C, Papin A, et al. Lymphoid-like environment, which promotes proliferation and induces resistance to BH3-Mimetics, is counteracted by Obinutuzumab in MCL: biological rationale for the oasis clinical trial. Blood. 2016;128:1096.
85. Kumar S, Vij R, Kaufman J, et al. Phase 1 study of Venetoclax monotherapy for relapsed/refractory multiple myeloma. In Haematologica. Ferrata Storti Foundation Via Giuseppe Belli 4, 27100 Pavia, Italy 2016:328–328.
86. Konopleva M, Pollyea DA, Potluri J, et al. Efficacy and biological correlates of response in a phase II study of Venetoclax monotherapy in patients with acute Myelogenous leukemia. Cancer Discov. 2016;6:1106–17.

Proteasome Inhibitors with a Focus on Bortezomib

Kevin Barley and Samir Parekh

Abstract Proteasome inhibitors have changed the treatment landscape for multiple myeloma and are being increasingly used in the treatment of lymphoma; however, patients eventually have progressive disease and development resistance to treatment. Multiple unique mechanisms of resistance have been identified, and they are unified by reducing a cell's sensitivity to endoplasmic reticulum stress either from changes intrinsic to the cancer cell or extrinsic to the cancer cell and due to changes in the microenvironment. These pathways primarily involve upregulation of proteasome subunits increasing the capacity to degrade unfolded proteins and plasmacytic differentiation to a more immature plasma cell phenotype with reduced immunoglobulin production. Understanding these mechanisms of resistance can inform therapeutic options to reverse drug resistance or use of novel combinations to synergistically target the unfolded protein response pathway.

Keywords Ubiquitin proteasome system · Proteasome inhibitors · Unfolded protein response · Plasmacytic differentiation

Abbreviations

ABC	Activated B-cell
ABCB1	ATP-binding cassette B1
ATF4	Activating transcription factor 4
ATF6	Activating transcription factor 6
BH	BCL-2 homology

BMMSC	Bone marrow mesenchymal stem cell
CYP26	Cytochrome P450 26
DLBCL	Diffuse large B-cell lymphoma
DRD2	Dopamine receptor D-2
E1	Ubiquitin activating enzyme
E2	Ubiquitin conjugating enzyme
E3	Terminal ubiquitin ligase
EGFR	Epidermal growth factor receptor
EIF2α	Eukaryotic Translation Initiation Factor 2α
ER	Endoplasmic reticulum
GCB	Germinal center B-cell
GCN2	EIF2α kinase 4
GLI	Glioma family transcription factors
GRP78	78-kDa glucose regulated protein
HDAC6	Histone deacetylase 6
Hh	Hedgehog pathway
HIV-1	Human immunodeficiency virus-1
HSP	Heat shock protein
Ig	Immunoglobulin
IKK	IκB kinase
IL-6	Interleukin-6
IRE1	Inositol requiring enzyme 1
IRF4	Interferon regulatory factor 4
ISR	Integrated stress response
JAK	Janus associated kinase
MCL	Mantle cell lymphoma
miR	microRNA
MM	Multiple myeloma
NFκB	Nuclear factor kappa B
NHL	Non-Hodgkin's lymphoma
PADI	Peptidyl arginine deaminase
PERK	EIF2α kinase 3
PI	Proteasome inhibitor
PSMB5	β5 subunit of the proteasome
PTCH1	Patched-1
SHH	Sonic hedgehog
SMO	Smoothened
STAT3	Signal transducer, and activator of transcription 3
TCL	T-cell lymphoma
TGF-β	Transforming growth factor β
TJP1	Tight junction protein 1
TNFα	tumor necrosis factor α
UPR	Unfolded protein response
XBP-1	X-box binding protein 1

Introduction

The ubiquitin proteasome system refers to the enzymes involved in the ubiquitination of target proteins and the proteasome, which is a multi-enzyme complex responsible for the protein degradation of many intracellular proteins in order to maintain protein homeostasis, clear misfolded proteins, and regulate proteins involved in signal transduction and regulation of the cell cycle. Since the FDA approval of the proteasome inhibitor (PI) bortezomib in 2003 for the treatment of multiple myeloma (MM), PIs have become increasingly important in the treatment of many subtypes of non-Hodgkin's lymphoma (NHL) including mantle cell lymphoma (MCL), follicular lymphoma, non-germinal center diffuse large B-cell lymphoma (DLBCL), and Waldenström's macroglobulinemia; however, the development of resistance to PIs is frequent [1–4]. A more detailed understanding of the mechanism of action and resistance of PIs is required to allow the development of tools to identify patients who will be resistant to PIs and the development of novel agents to overcome resistance. Second generation and oral PIs are now available; however, this chapter will focus on the mechanisms of resistance to bortezomib. Although this book focuses primarily on lymphoma, since PIs were first developed in MM and the majority of research into the mechanisms of resistance has been in MM, in this chapter, we will discuss resistance mechanisms drawing from data in both lymphomas and MM.

The Ubiquitin Proteasome System

Protein degradation occurs in a cascade involving an ubiquitin activating enzyme (E1), a ubiquitin conjugating enzyme (E2), and a terminal ubiquitin ligase (E3). In an ATP-dependent manner, ubiquitin is activated by its transfer to an E1 enzyme. Subsequently, the ubiquitin molecule is transferred to the active cysteine site of an E2 enzyme. Finally, an E3 ubiquitin ligase facilitates the transfer of the ubiquitin from the E2 enzyme to the protein targeted for degradation. Ubiquitin is most commonly transferred to an amino group of a lysine residue of the target protein or to the amino terminus of the peptide. This process is repeated several times with additional ubiquitin molecules transferred to lysine residues of the previously transferred ubiquitin. Upon polyubiquitination by 4–5 ubiquitin molecules, the protein is targeted to the 26S proteasome for degradation. In humans, there are 2 E1 ubiquitin enzymes (UBA1, UBA6), approximately 30 E2 enzymes, and hundreds of E3 ligases, and, therefore, the specificity of the ubiquitin proteasome system is primarily a function of the E3 ubiquitin ligases [5].

The 26S proteasome is a large cylindrical protein formed from a 20S catalytic core particle with 19S regulatory subunits capped on both ends. The 20S core particle is comprised of 4 stacked rings, 2 outer α-rings and 2 inner β-rings. The α-rings of the core particle serve as a gate to prevent the entrance of substrates not targeted by ubiquitin from entering the complex. The β-rings are composed of 7 subunits (β1–7), three of which have a unique proteolytic activity: peptidyl-glutamyl-hydrolyzing or caspase-like (β1), trypsin-like (β2), and chymotrypsin-like (β5). After a protein is polyubiquitinated, the ubiquitin chain is recognized by the lid-like structure of the 19S subunit, the ubiquitin chain is removed, and the protein is denatured by the ATPases at the base of the 19S subunit and then degraded by the proteolytic activity of the 20S proteasome [6]. There is a similar and related proteasome system, the immunoproteasome, which is more prevalent in hematopoietic cells. It differs from the conventional proteasome primarily by alternate β subunits, with $β1_i$, $β2_i$, and $β5_i$, in place of β1, β2, and β5, which have slightly different structures but similar enzymatic activity [7].

Proteasome Inhibitors: Mechanism of Anti-tumor Effect

Bortezomib, the first clinically active PI, is a dipeptide boronic acid analog that reversibly inhibits the 20S proteasome at the chymotryptic site [8, 9]. Carfilzomib, a second generation PI, is a tetrapeptide epoxyketone analog of epoxomicin, which binds irreversibly to the chymotryptic subunit of the 20S proteasome, and at higher doses is able to bind to the trypsin-like subunit. Carfilzomib also has less inhibition of off-target proteases than bortezomib [10]. Ixazomib is an orally bioavailable boronic acid derivative that is a pro-drug which is rapidly hydrolyzed to MLN2238, the active PI. Similar to carfilzomib, it inhibits the chymotryptic subunit of the proteasome and to a lesser degree the trypsin-like subunit [11]. All of these proteasome inhibitors have a similar activity against the immunoproteasome and the conventional proteasome [7]. Owing to the numerous proteins and pathways regulated and degraded by the proteasome, inhibiting the proteasome has numerous effects on both cancer cells and the normal cells that comprise the cancer's microenvironment. The initial proposed mechanism of PI's anti-myeloma and anti-lymphoma effects was the inhibitory effect on the transcription factor nuclear factor kappa B (NFκB); however, further studies showed that the mechanism relies on activating and dysregulating the unfolded protein response (UPR) and upregulation of the proapoptotic protein NOXA (Fig. 1). Lymphoma and MM cells are highly dependent upon the function of UPR, and PIs not only lead to rapid protein accumulation to trigger the UPR but also dysregulate it, promoting apoptosis.

Early in its development, bortezomib was shown to inhibit the NFκB pathway, an important pathway for tumor survival and proliferation in lymphoma. In the canonical NFκB pathway, NFκB is negatively regulated by IκB, which binds to NFκB preventing translocation to the nucleus where it acts as a transcription factor. IκB is in turn negatively regulated by a number of proteins and cytokines that lead to the phosphorylation of IκB by the IκB kinase (IKK), which leads to the polyubiquitination and proteasomal degradation of IκB [12]. Proteasome inhibition leads to the accumulation of IκB, which results in increased inhibition of NFκB.

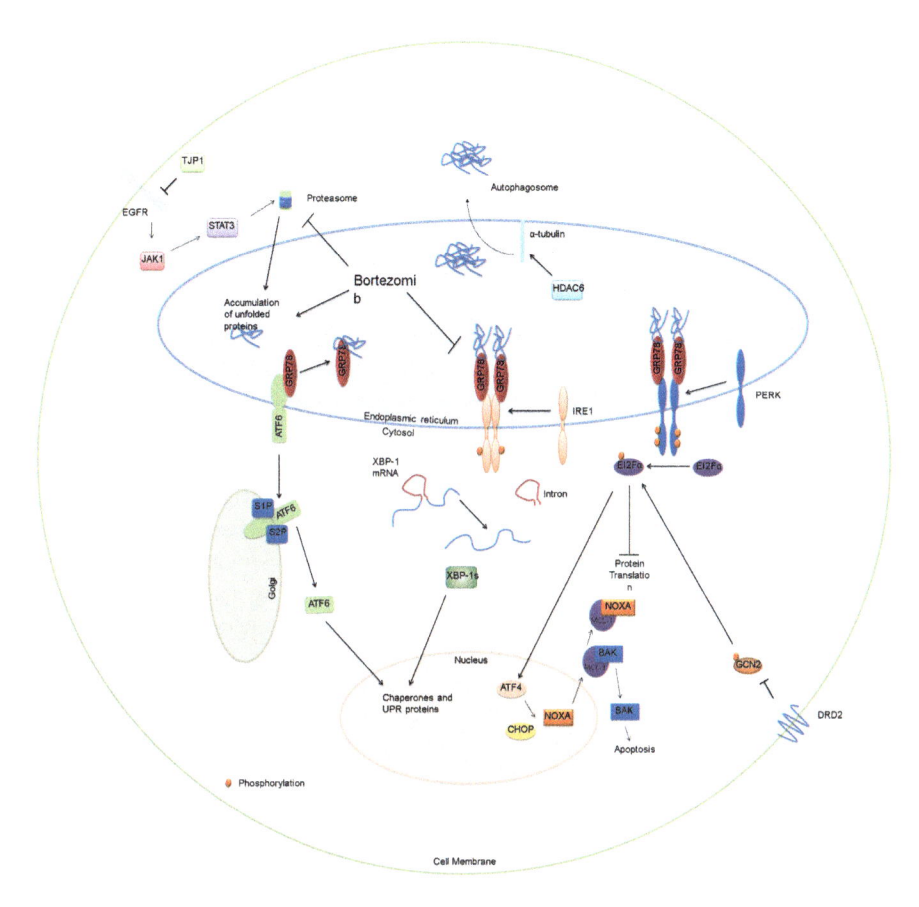

Fig. 1 The unfolded protein response. Bortezomib inhibits the proteasome leading to accumulation of unfolded/misfolded proteins. These proteins are recognized by GRP78, which releases ATF6. ATF6 is cleaved by S1P and S2P in the Golgi and translocates to the nucleus to upregulate chaperones and UPR proteins. IRE1 recognizes GRP78, oligomerizes and undergoes autophosphorylation, and this is inhibited by bortezomib. The active IRE1 splices XBP-1, which leads to translation of chaperones and UPR proteins. PERK also oligomerizes and autophosphorylates leading to activation of EI2Fα which inhibits protein translation. Prolonged activation of the EI2Fα leads to upregulation of ATF4 and subsequently CHOP and NOXA. NOXA displaces BAK from MCL-1 leading to apoptosis. HDAC6 can deacetylate α-tubulin, which upregulates autophagy. EGFR can signal through JAK1 and STAT3 to upregulate translation of proteasome subunits, and this pathway is inhibited by TJP1. GNC2 is also able to activate EIF2α, which is prevented by signaling through DRD2

Gene expression profiling of MM patients responding to bortezomib confirmed the inhibition of this pathway with bortezomib treatment, but this study was not structured to determine if these changes were a cause or an effect of apoptosis [13]. In contrast, in vitro studies using a direct IKK inhibitor in MM cells resulted in decreased IκB phosphorylation, increased levels of IκB, decreased tumor necrosis factor α (TNFα)-inducible activity of NFκB, and growth arrest at G_1, but it did not induce apoptosis. In the same experiment, treatment with bortezomib resulted in similar changes to the NFκB pathway but was cytotoxic to MM cells resulting in apoptosis [12]. This suggests that the NFκB pathway may be active in MM and lymphoma and a potential target, but that this pathway alone was inadequate to explain the cytotoxicity of bortezomib, and it did not evaluate the constitutive activity of the NFκB pathway. Further studies by the same group showed that bortezomib actually also activates IKK and RIP2 which over time lead to phosphorylation and degradation of IκB and resultant increased constitutive activation of NFκB, but this did not negatively impact the cytotoxic effect of bortezomib. The addition of a specific IKK inhibitor resulted in increased cytotoxicity [14]. These results further suggest that the NFκB pathway is an important target in MM and lymphoma, but it is not the mechanism of proteasome inhibitors activity.

The unfolded protein response is an important signaling pathway in lymphoma and MM cells. Plasma cells have a highly developed endoplasmic reticulum (ER) and system of chaperones enabling the production of large quantities of immunoglobulin (Ig). Upon accumulation of unfolded or misfolded proteins in the ER, there is stress to the ER triggering the UPR signaling pathway to restore homeostasis, or, failing that, apoptosis. A functional UPR is necessary for plasma cells, and activation of B cells lacking proteins in the UPR fails to lead to the differentiation into plasma cells [15]. Activation of the UPR results in signals to temporarily reduce protein translation, increases production of chaperones to increase protein folding, trafficking of proteins from the ER to the proteasome for degradation, and, if homeostasis is not restored, ultimately this will lead to apoptosis. During folding, proteins are glycosylated, and misfolded proteins are recognized by this lack of glycosylation by 78-kDa glucose regulated protein (GRP78), a heat shock protein (HSP) 70 family member. GRP78 is bound to the activating transcription factor 6 (ATF6) on the ER membrane and dissociates from ATF6 upon recognition of unglycosylated proteins. Binding of GRP78 to unfolded proteins and oligomerization triggers three pathways in the UPR: ATF6, Eukaryotic Translation Initiation Factor 2 α (EIF2α) Kinase 3 (PERK), and inositol requiring enzyme 1 (IRE1) [16]. ATF6 having been released from GRP78 translocates to the Golgi apparatus and is cleaved by the proteases S1P and S2P to its active form. The active cleaved ATF6 translocates to the nucleus to increase production of proteins involved in protein folding and clearance of unfolded proteins including GRP78 [17]. PERK binds to GRP78 and oligomerization results in autophosphorylation and activation. Activated PERK phosphorylates EIF2α leading to a generalized attenuation of translation and cell cycle arrest in G1 [15, 18]. Prolonged activation of PERK results in selective translation of the pro-apoptotic transcription factor ATF4. ATF4 transcriptionally upregulates pro-apoptotic proteins CHOP and the BCL-2 family protein NOXA [19, 20]. Similar to PERK, IRE1 oligomerizes and undergoes autophosphorylation allowing its endoribonuclease to excise an intron from the transcription factor X-box binding protein 1 (XBP-1). After translation, the active spliced XBP-1 translocates to the nucleus to increase production of proteins involved in protein folding and clearance of unfolded proteins [15, 18]. The three arms of the UPR are activated simultaneously, and the transition from anti-apoptotic IRE1 and ATF6 to pro-apoptotic PERK is not due to preferential signaling of one of the pathways in normal physiological states, but instead to the relative timing of activation of the signaling cascades with PERK activation of ATF4 being a delayed event, which ultimately results in the translation of pro-apoptotic proteins, in particular NOXA [18].

The BCL-2 family proteins are important regulators of apoptosis that share one or more of four BCL-2 homology (BH) domains, BH1, BH2, BH3, and BH4. NOXA is a BCL-2 family member that contains only a single BH3 domain and is a pro-apoptotic regulatory protein. MCL-1 functions by binding BAK and, thereby, preventing the cascade of oligomerization of BAK which leads to mitochondrial outer membrane permeabilization causing apoptosis [21]. NOXA inhibits the anti-apoptotic MCL-1 by binding to MCL-1 releasing BAK, thereby promoting apoptosis. In MM and lymphoma cell lines, exposure to bortezomib resulted in increased mRNA and protein expression of NOXA, which results in release of BAK from MCL-1, caspase cleavage and apoptosis, and inhibition of NOXA with interfering RNA, reverses the cytotoxicity of bortezomib [19, 22–27]. NOXA expression after bortezomib exposure is upregulated by ATF3 and ATF4, which have been shown to form a complex that directly binds to the NOXA promoter. Inhibition of ATF4 inhibits bortezomib-induced NOXA overexpression, but inhibition of ATF3 only partially inhibits NOXA overexpression [19, 20]. Thus, bortezomib induces the UPR, which results in the upregulation of ATF3 and ATF4, and ultimately leads to NOXA upregulation, which disrupts the inhibitory interaction between MCL-1 and BAK allowing BAK to induce apoptosis.

In addition to stimulating the UPR, PIs also dysregulate the UPR. In MM cells treated with inducers of ER stress, the UPR is activated and there is increased expression of spliced XBP-1, as expected; however, this increased expression of spliced XBP-1 is not seen in bortezomib treated cells suggesting that bortezomib not only induces ER stress but also impairs the UPR shifting it towards the pro-apoptotic pathways [28]. As cells are exposed to increasing concentrations of PIs, there is reduced expression of spliced XBP-1 which is correlated with the induction of apoptosis and suggests that this dysregulation of the UPR is an important mechanism of its cytotoxicity [15]. By a mechanism that is not fully elucidated, bortezomib inhibits the initial autophosphorylation step of the IRE1/XBP-1 arm of the UPR, thereby preventing the splicing of XBP-1; however, this does not prevent the activation of the pro-apoptotic functions of the UPR via PERK. In summary, lymphoma and MM cells are dependent upon a functioning UPR, and treatment with PIs not only induces ER stress to activate the UPR, but also impairs the function of the UPR by preventing IRE1 activation and splicing of XBP-1. This results in the transcriptional upregulation of NOXA, which displaces MCL-1 from BAK resulting in the induction of apoptosis [29].

Cell Intrinsic Mechanisms of Resistance

There are multiple mechanisms postulated to explain bortezomib resistance in lymphomas and MM. These mechanisms can be broadly categorized into genetic or physiologic changes that are intrinsic to the malignant lymphoma or MM cell and to alterations that are extrinsic to the malignant cell and, instead, involve changes to the microenvironment.

Proteasome Subunit Mutations

The proteasome inhibitory activity of PIs is dependent upon binding to the β5 subunit of the proteasome (PSMB5). In PI resistance models developed from tumor cell lines with a long exposure to PIs, mutations in PSMB5 are frequently observed [30–32]. Multiple mutations have been observed in different cell lines, but the majority involve amino acid positions 45–52 and have been shown to impair binding of multiple PIs to PSMB5 and inhibit proteasome activity, in vitro [33, 34]. The different mutations have a varying impact on the proteasome inhibitory effect of PIs with A49V having the most significant inhibitory effect [35]. The PSMB5 mutations may not be the only mechanism of drug resistance present in these in vitro models, as transfection of PSMB5 A49V mutations into untreated cell lines results in a significantly lesser degree of PI resistance [30]. Despite the high frequency of PSMB5 mutations in in vitro models, these mutations have not been reported in patients with resistance to PIs [36–39]. Thus, while PSMB5 mutations are frequently found in cell culture based models of PI resistance, they are unlikely to be an important mechanism of PI resistance for patients. These data also highlight the potential differences in in vitro resistance models in which cells are exposed to chronic low doses of PIs and in vivo resistance in which resistance is either present prior to exposure or develops while receiving intermittent exposure to higher doses of PIs.

Efflux Pumps

Efflux pumps are an important mechanism of drug resistance to a variety of chemotherapeutic agents [40]. The multidrug efflux pump P-glycoprotein (PGP), also referred to as ATP-binding cassette B1 (ABCB1), has been implicated in PI resistance. It is important to note that PGP is degraded by the proteasome, and inhibition of the proteasome leads to increased concentrations of PGP which does not necessarily reflect PI resistance [41]. Early studies raised doubts about whether bortezomib was a substrate for PGP, and thus, whether increased PGP expression could affect sensitivity to bortezomib. In a cell culture study using cell lines that overexpressed PGP and other lines overexpressing other efflux pumps, increased PGP expression conferred a mild degree of resistance, and sensitivity was unaffected by the other efflux pumps tested [42]. Similarly, in a MM model with cells overexpressing PGP, ultrahigh performance liquid chromatography-mass spectrometry found significantly lower intracellular concentrations of bortezomib at high PGP concentrations and reduced sensitivity to bortezomib. However, the expression of PGP required to reduce bortezomib concentrations was very high and, the authors argued, was unlikely to be of clinical significance [43]. Another study using cell lines found only mild resistance with bortezomib in cell lines overexpressing PGP compared to controls. However, the second generation PI carfilzomib had a high degree of resistance associated with PGP expression, and blocking PGP restored sensitivity to carfilzomib in the resistant cells [32]. In PI resistance models developed from tumor cell lines with a long exposure to PIs, PGP is not differentially expressed in bortezomib-resistant versus bortezomib-sensitive cells; however, in carfilzomib-resistant cells, PGP was one of the most highly overexpressed proteins [34]. There have also not been any reports in patients exposed to PIs suggesting that resistance was associated with increased PGP expression; however, these studies require an additional biopsy at the time of progression, and there is insufficient data in the literature. Thus, high expression of PGP may be able to cause a mild degree of bortezomib resistance, but this has not been shown to be a clinically relevant mechanism of bortezomib resistance in vitro or in vivo. Importantly, this is not a class effect, and there is evidence that carfilzomib is effluxed through PGP, so whether PGP or other efflux pumps are a cause of resistance will need to be evaluated for each PI individually.

Autophagy

Autophagy is a process by which aggresomes engulf proteins and other molecules and traffic them to lysosomes for degradation. Autophagy had been thought of as a non-selective degradation pathway; however, evidence has accumulated showing that molecules are targeted for autophagy in a similar way as they are to the ubiquitin proteasome system, and that there is cross-talk between these two systems [44]. PIs are able to lead to the activation of the UPR and impair its ability to restore homeostasis via inhibition of XBP-1 splicing, which leads to further protein accumulation in the ER. In response, autophagy can be activated and the proteins can be targeted to aggresomes and ultimately to lysosomes for degradation [45]. Subsequent to activation by PERK in the UPR, ATF4 is able to stimulate autophagy and this activation is more pronounced when cells are also treated with PIs [46, 47]. In DLBCL cell lines, bortezomib induced autophagy in a dose-dependent manner and was associated with partial resistance to bortezomib. The addition of an autophagy inhibitor to bortezomib enhanced the cytotoxicity in DLBCL. In the same study, bortezomib was not active in a follicular lymphoma cell line unless an autophagy inhibitor was also given [48]. The autophagy system is dependent upon histone deacetylase 6 (HDAC6) epigenetic mediated expression of several proteins as well deacetylation of UPR proteins such as α–tubulin, which results in stimulation of autophagy [45–48]. Dual inhibition with histone deacetylase inhibitors is synergistic both in preclinical models and in patients with MM [49, 50]. An in vitro study of the combination of an HDAC6 inhibitor and bortezomib in different subtypes of lymphoma including activated B-cell (ABC) DLBCL, germinal center B-cell (GCB) DLBCL, MCL, and T-lymphoma found synergy between the two agents. In an analysis of patient samples with different subtypes of lymphoma, they also found that more aggressive lymphomas (DLBCL, MCL, TCL) compared to more indolent lymphomas had higher expression of UPR proteins such as GRP78 and XBP-1 suggesting a greater dependence upon the UPR pathway in more activated and differentiated lymphomas [51].

Plasmacytic Differentiation

The process of lymphocyte activation and differentiation into plasma cells involves several steps, each with associated gene expression changes. In particular, the transcriptional repressor PRDM1 is expressed early in differentiation, and XBP-1 is expressed late in differentiation as Igs begin to be synthesized in large quantities. Without this increased expression of XBP-1 and associated increased efficiency of the UPR pathway, differentiation will halt, and the lymphocytes and plasma cells that survive produce fewer Ig [52, 53]. Alterations in gene expression consistent with transition to an immature undifferentiated plasma cell have been implicated in PI resistance. In a model of bortezomib-resistant MCL, resistant MCL cells developed a plasmacytic differentiation signature similar to an early plasma cell with expression of PRDM1 and low expression of XBP-1. Consistent with the low XBP-1 expression in resistant cells, there was very low Ig excretion in the bortezomib resistant cell lines. As the MCL cells developed an early plasmacytic differentiation phenotype, a dependence on interferon regulatory factor 4 (IRF4) developed, and knockdown of IRF4 was cytotoxic [54]. Of note, IRF4 is downstream of the target of thalidomide, lenalidomide, and pomalidomide, suggesting that as resistance to PIs develops in MCL, a dependence upon the target of, and, therefore sensitivity to lenalidomide develops [55, 56]. The model of resistance developed in this study is that as lymphoma cells develop resistance to PIs they develop plasmacytic differentiation with the associated more efficient UPR and proteasome capacity but without activating secretion of Ig; in contrast, myeloma cells developing resistance dedifferentiate to an early plasma cell reducing the production of immunoglobulin and associated proteasome load while maintaining or enhancing the efficiency of the UPR and proteasome capacity.

This plasmacytic differentiation model of PI resistance in which there is a shifting balance in the proteasome load versus proteasome capacity was first conceived of in studying PI resistance in MM. Early on it was recognized that the degree of Ig synthesis correlated with PI sensitivity, which suggests that the amount of protein the proteasome may need to degrade, or, similarly, the degree of stimulus activating the UPR correlated with PI sensitivity [57, 58]. In a comparison of PI sensitive and resistant MM cell lines, sensitive cells were found to have increased proteasomal protein degradation (increased proteasome load). They also found that other PI sensitive MM cell lines had reduced expression of proteasome catalytic subunits and activity (reduced proteasome capacity) and inducing β subunit expression promoted PI resistance [59]. In MM cell lines exposed to bortezomib as well as pretreatment patient samples, resistance was associated with reduced expression of the UPR proteins IRE1 and XBP-1 [60–62]. This study also found that IRE1 and XBP-1 suppressed MM cells had an immunophenotype consistent with a less well differentiated plasma cell. The patient samples responsive to bortezomib had a gene expression profile consistent with a mature plasma cell, whereas the resistant MM cells were less well differentiated [60].

Proteasome Subunit Expression

Recently, a novel mechanism of resistance involving tight junction protein 1 (TJP1) was suggested. Multiple clinical trials of bortezomib were used to identify responders and non-responders to bortezomib, and their gene expression profiles were analyzed to find aberrantly expressed genes with confirmation in a separate data set. TJP1 was highly underexpressed in MM cells from bortezomib resistant patients. TJP1 had not previously been studied in myeloma and is important in tight junction formation. The investigators then created TJP1 knockdown MM cell lines and confirmed that absence of TJP1 conferred PI resistance and overexpression of TJP1 in PI resistant MM cell lines restored sensitivity. This was replicated in MCL cell lines with the same results. The expression of TJP1 was inversely correlated with the immunoproteasome subunits $\beta 1_i$ and $\beta 5_i$ and proteasome activity, and the overexpression and knockdown of $\beta 1_i$ and $\beta 5_i$, was sufficient to recapitulate bortezomib resistance and sensitivity, respectively. A series of experiments yielded a model in which TJP1 inhibited a signaling cascade involving the epidermal growth factor receptor (EGFR), Janus associated kinase (JAK) and signal transducer, and activator of transcription 3 (STAT3), and the activation of this pathway by suppression of TJP1 increased expression of the $\beta 1_i$ and $\beta 5_i$ subunits. In line with this implicated pathway, it was shown that exposure to EGFR inhibitors reduced EGFR signaling, expression of the $\beta 1_i$ and $\beta 5_i$ subunits, and increased sensitivity to bortezomib [63]. In support of this model, a separate group simultaneously reported that a novel STAT3 inhibitor had mild anti-MM activity, but, more importantly, restored bortezomib-sensitivity to MM in resistant MM cell lines. As these experiments were performed at approximately the same time by separate groups, TJP1 expression was not explored in this study [64].

BCL-2

MM cells are particularly dependent upon MCL-1 expression; however, some MM cells are more dependent upon BCL-2 and BCL-XL to inhibit apoptosis. Similarly, different lymphomas have a differential dependence upon BCL-2, MCL-1, and BCL-XL [65]. In lymphoma cell lines, bortezomib induced apoptosis was inhibited with BCL-2 overexpression and enhanced with a BCL-2 inhibitor [66]. This suggests alterations in the relative expression of various BCL-2 family members may contribute to PI resistance.

In summary, there are multiple potential cell intrinsic mechanisms of resistance to PIs in lymphoma, but the most important mechanism is likely related to a balance between the demand on the proteasome (proteasome load) and the capacity for the proteasome to meet this demand. There are multiple factors that affect this balance between proteasome load and capacity; importantly, as lymphocytes differentiate into activated B-cells and early undifferentiated plasma cells, the proteasome capacity increases without an increase in proteasome load leading to PI resistance. The well-differentiated plasma cell has an increased proteasome capacity but also significantly increased proteasome load leading to PI sensitivity. Thus, well differentiated plasma cells in MM can dedifferentiate to a less Ig secreting plasma cell to acquire resistance, and lymphoma cells are able to differentiate into an immature plasma cell to acquire PI resistance. Similarly, as was shown in bortezomib-treated patients with MM, PI resistance was associated with an increase in proteasome formation by decreased expression of TJP1 and induction of the EGFR/JAK/STAT3 pathway leading to increased expression of immunoproteasome subunits. Finally, autophagy, functioning as a complementary protein degradation system, is able to degrade a portion of the proteasome load, particularly under times of ER stress when the autophagy system is activated. Thus, increased dependence upon the autophagy system can, in effect, increase the proteasome capacity contributing to PI resistance.

Cell Extrinsic Mechanisms of Resistance

The tumor microenvironment plays a critical role in tumor survival during treatment and at relapse in MM and lymphoma [67–70]. There are multiple pathways by which the microenvironment supports MM and lymphoma cells including induction of immune tolerance and promotion of angiogenesis, but also by paracrine signaling between the microenvironment and tumor cells that promotes drug resistance. In MM, bone marrow mesenchymal stem cells (BMMSCs) have a distinct genomic profile in comparison to that of normal controls. This abnormal phenotype of MM BMMSCs is not due to the presence of a common progenitor for the MM plasma cells and BMMSCs, as cytogenetic abnormalities found in the plasma cells are not found in the BMMSCs [71]. However, the abnormal transcriptional profile persists even when BMMSCs are cultured in the absence of MM cells, which suggests that there is a genetic or epigenetic alteration in the microenvironment itself [72, 73].

Interleukin-6

Interleukin-6 (IL-6), which is secreted primarily by bone marrow mesenchymal stem cells and macrophages in the microenvironment, is an important driver of proliferation and regulator of plasmacytic differentiation [74]. Peptidyl arginine deaminase (PADI) 2, an epigenetic modifier, was found to be highly significantly overexpressed in MM BMMSCs and, through histone deamination, was shown to be responsible for IL-6 production [74]. Coculture of PADI2-expressing BMMSCs with a MM cell line resulted in bortezomib resistance, which is consistent with the preclinical synergy seen with bortezomib and IL-6 blockade [75]. The mechanism of IL-6 mediated bortezomib resistance has not been fully elucidated, but IL-6 exposure leads to proliferation specifically of CD45+ plasma cells, which have a more immature immunophenotype. This suggests the microenvironment may be involved in the promoting plasmacytic dedifferentiation, and, thereby, leads to bortezomib resistance [76]. Additionally, IL-6 induces JAK/STAT3 signaling and increases MCL-1 expression, which may also contribute to bortezomib resistance [77, 78]. These effects may be mediated by microRNA (miR), which are small non-coding RNA that suppress RNA translationally or by mRNA degradation. Cell culture studies have shown that, via JAK/STAT signaling, IL-6 leads to upregulation of miR-21 and suppression of miR-15a. Suppression of miR-15a resulted in bortezomib resistance, and studies in CLL have found that BCL-2 is a target of miR-15a, so suppression miR-15a may increase expression of BCL-2 resulting in less MCL-1 dependence and bortezomib resistance [79–82]. In contrast, the elevated levels of miR-21 were found to support MM cell survival in the presence of bortezomib, and miR-21 inhibition was synergistic with bortezomib [83]. These findings were confirmed in a second study; however, the effects of miR-21 inhibition were only seen in cell lines with high baseline levels of miR-21. In addition to the paracrine cytokine signaling between BMMSCs [84] and plasma cells, BMMSCs are able to release exosomes containing miR. Isolating BMMSC derived exosomes and culturing MM cell lines with them results in increased survival and drug resistance, including PI resistance [85]. Similar studies in MCL have found that microenvironment-secreted IL-6 supports MCL survival and promotes resistance to bortezomib, and that this signaling is through the JAK/STAT pathway [86].

The Hedgehog Pathway

The hedgehog pathway (Hh) is a complex signaling pathway, which can act in both autocrine and paracrine ways. In the canonical pathway, the Hh ligand, most important of which is sonic hedgehog (SHH), is secreted from the cell. It binds to the receptor patched-1 (PTCH1), which releases the inhibition of smoothened (SMO). SMO accumulation results in nuclear localization and activation of glioma family transcription factors (GLI) [87]. In MM, plasma cells express SHH, and activation of the Hh pathway supports cell survival and promotes bortezomib resistance in cell lines grown with bone marrow stroma resulting in an immature plasma cell phenotype [87, 88]. Blockade of Hh signaling with a microenvironment SMO knockout resulted in restoration of plasma cell differentiation and sensitivity to bortezomib, which suggests paracrine signaling between MM cell derived SHH and microenvironment PTCH1 and SMO. SHH signaling in the microenvironment is able to upregulate cytochrome P450 26 (CYP26), a retinoid inactivating enzyme. In support of CYP26 as a target of SMO responsible for bortezomib resistance, coculture of MM cells, stroma, and a CYP26 resistant retinoid restores a mature plasma cell phenotype and bortezomib sensitivity. Similarly, in the SMO knockout, overexpression of CYP26 with lentiviral transfection resulted in an immature plasma cell phenotype and bortezomib resistance [88]. In summary, these studies suggest a bidirectional cross-talk between MM cells and the bone marrow microenvironment. MM cells secrete SHH, which signals through PTCH1 and SMO on the bone marrow stromal cells and leads to CYP26 overexpression. This results in degradation of retinoids in the microenvironment, preventing retinoic acid signaling to the MM cells, and resulting in dedifferentiation to an immature plasma cell phenotype, which is resistant to bortezomib.

Overcoming Bortezomib Resistance

The multiple modes of drug resistance to PIs in lymphoma offer multiple potential therapeutic options to overcome resistance. A central feature of many of the mechanisms of PI resistance in lymphoma is alterations in the balance of proteasome capacity and proteasome demand, which, for many of these mechanisms, is accomplished by differentiation in to an immature plasma cell phenotype. While many of the mechanisms of PI resistance converge on plasmacytic differentiation, they offer unique pathways for overcoming resistance, which can be grouped by the targeted pathways: targeting prosurvival factors the immature plasma cell is dependent upon, inducing differentiation into a mature plasma cell phenotype with X-BP1 expression and increased Ig secretion, enhancing the activation of the unfolded protein response, and targeting BCL-2 family proteins (Table 1).

Targeting the Immature Plasma Cell

Differentiation from a B-cell to a plasma cell requires many transcription factors, including X-BP1 and IRF4. X-BP1 is critical in the final stages of differentiation and IRF4 is critical at the stage of an immature plasma cell. MCL cells develop PI resistance by differentiating in to an immature plasma cell and simultaneously develop dependence upon IRF4 such that IRF4 inhibition is cytotoxic [54, 89].

Table 1 Overcoming bortezomib resistance

Pathway	Drug/target
Targeting the immature plasma cell	IRF4; lenalidomide
Differentiation induction	Inhibition of Interleukin-6; siltuximab

	Hh pathway inhibition
	  SMO inhibitors; vismodegib, sonidegib
	  GlI inhibitors; arsenic trioxide
	  SHH inhibitors
	  Retinoids

Enhancing activation of the UPR	Autophagy inhibition
	  HSP90 inhibitors
	  TGF-β inhibitors

	TJP1 pathway inhibition; erlotinib
	S1P, S2P inhibition; nelfinavir
	DRD2 inhibition; ONC201
BCL-2 inhibition	Venetoclax

Lenalidomide binds to the E3 ubiquitin ligase cereblon resulting in degradation of the transcription factors ikaros and aiolos. IRF4 is a transcriptional target of ikaros and aiolos, so IRF4 is able to be targeted with lenalidomide. As such, when PI resistance develops due to plasmacytic differentiation, the cells are dependent upon IRF4 and able to be targeted with lenalidomide. Lenalidomide is known to have activity in MCL, and this understanding of the mechanism of bortezomib resistance raises the possibility or either combination therapy with PIs and lenalidomide or sequencing therapy to induce lenalidomide sensitivity with initial treatment with bortezomib. This is not based upon the typical model of synergy in which one or both drugs potentiate the action of the other. Instead, similar to seen with combination of certain antibiotics in resistant infections, there is a "seesaw effect" in which the development of resistance to one drug induces sensitivity to the other drug [90].

Differentiation Induction

It may be possible to reverse the bortezomib resistance due to an immature plasma cell phenotype by promoting differentiation into a more mature plasma cell. In both MM and MCL, IL-6 signaling by the tumor microenvironment is able to induce differentiation to an immature plasma cell phenotype and to lead to bortezomib resistance [76, 86]. IL-6 is able to be targeted with monoclonal antibodies including tocilizumab and siltuximab which are FDA approved for other indications. In preclinical models, IL-6 inhibition has demonstrated synergy with bortezomib [75]. Siltuximab has been studied in multiple clinical trials in MM. Small studies evaluating siltuximab as monotherapy found very limited responses [91, 92]. There are two trials of a bortezomib-based regimen with or without siltuximab [93, 94]. Both studies failed to meet their primary endpoints but also had a suggestion of potential benefit. One study found a significant benefit in progression free survival in patients treated in the United States and Western Europe but not other locations for unclear reasons. The other study found statistically significantly higher response rates to very good partial response or better but not to complete response rate, which was the primary end point. These studies have not proven a benefit to IL-6 blockade in overcoming bortezomib resistance, but suggest it warrants further study. An important consideration is that these trials included patients regardless of IL-6 levels. As there are multiple mechanisms of bortezomib resistance, it's possible that IL-6 may be an important mechanism in a limited number of patients, and, therefore, that IL-6 blockade may only be beneficial in this subset of patients. It's possible anti-IL-6 therapy may be beneficial in the subset of patients with high IL-6 levels or in patients, who, at time of progression on PIs, have elevated IL-6 levels. The Hh pathway is also an important driver of differentiation to an immature plasma cell phenotype and bortezomib resistance, and preclinical data suggest Hh inhibition restores sensitivity [88]. Signaling between the tumor and microenvironment via the Hh pathway results in upregulation of CYP26, which degrades retinoids involved in the terminal differentiation of plasma cells. This activation of the Hh pathway results in bortezomib resistance. There are multiple potential therapeutic targets within the Hh pathway. Sonidegib and vismodegib are SMO inhibitors, which are FDA approved for the treatment of basal cell carcinoma. Their use is potentially limited by significant toxicity; however, clinical trials evaluating vismodegib in lymphoma and MM are ongoing [95]. The transcription factor GLI is the downstream target of the Hh pathway and can be inhibited by direct GLI inhibitors which are under development as well as by arsenic trioxide [96, 97]. Arsenic trioxide has been studied in a few small trials in MM, and, as monotherapy, has very limited efficacy, but more promising efficacy is seen in combination with bortezomib [98–100]. These studies have included patients with and without prior bortezomib exposure and were not designed to clearly evaluate whether the mechanism of action was related to bortezomib resistance. Inhibitors of SHH are under development, but are not in human trials at this time. Finally, as the mechanism of the Hh pathway is related to induction of CYP26 and inhibition of retinoid-induced differentiation into a mature plasma cell phenotype, both retinoids and inhibitors of CYP26 offer the potential to inhibit this resistance pathway. Multiple inhibitors of CYP26 have been synthesized, but they are early in development, and preclinical data in lymphoma and MM are not yet available, but may be therapeutic options in the future [101]. Retinoids that are not able to be metabolized by CYP26 have also been developed, and, in preclinical models, are able to overcome bortezomib resistance [88]. Although ATRA metabolized by CYP26, pharmacologic dosing of ATRA may be at concentrations that are able to induce plasma cell differentiation despite CYP26. Supporting this, in preclinical models, ATRA is able to induce a mature plasma cell phenotype and bortezomib sensitivity in MM cells [58].

Synergistically Activating the Unfolded Protein Response

Activation and dysregulation of the UPR is the primary mechanism of action of bortezomib, and many mechanisms of resistance are the result of cellular changes that impair the ability of bortezomib to induce the UPR or increase the cell's tolerance to ER stress. The autophagy system has multiple potential targets. HDACs, in particular HDAC6, are important for maintaining and activating the autophagy system, which is able to degrade misfolded proteins when the proteasome is inhibited. The pan-HDAC inhibitor panobinostat is active in MM and FDA approved for use in combination with bortezomib [49, 50]. Preclinical studies in a variety of lymphomas have evaluated multiple HDAC inhibitors and found both synergy with PIs and the ability to overcome PI resistance, and they are now being tested clinically [51, 102–105]. As the autophagy system is activated when GRP78 oligomerizes leading to autophosphorylation of PERK and increased expression of ATF4, inhibition of GRP78 could impair autophagy. HSP90 acts to stabilize GRP78 preventing activation of the UPR, and, in a preclinical MCL model, an HSP90 inhibitor was synergistic with bortezomib and able to overcome bortezomib resistance [106]. Autophagy is also inducible by transforming growth factor β (TGF-β). In MM cell lines, a TGF-β inhibitor was able to bock the induction of autophagy, have a synergistic anti-MM effect with bortezomib, and overcome bortezomib resistance [107]. An important mechanism of bortezomib resistance is reduced expression of TJP-1 which results in upregulation of proteasome subunit translation [63]. TJP-1 suppression results in activation of an EGFR, JAK, STAT3 pathway, and in preclinical models, inhibition of this pathway with the EGFR inhibitor, erlotinib, was able to overcome bortezomib resistance. Targeting EGFR, JAK or STAT3 has not been clinically evaluated in lymphoma or MM but are a potential route to overcoming bortezomib resistance with currently available drugs. Nelfinavir is an FDA approved human immunodeficiency virus-1 (HIV-1) protease inhibitor, which is able to act synergistically with PIs. Nelfinavir is able to induce the UPR, but it also inhibits the phosphatases S1P and S2P, which activate the prosurvival ATF6 [108–111]. Thus, as bortezomib activates the UPR but inhibits one of the prosurvival pathways, IRE1, nelfinavir also activates the UPR and inhibits the prosurvival ATF6 pathway, providing potential synergy and the ability to overcome resistance. In MM, nelfinavir has been tested in combination with bortezomib in phase I and II studies with impressive results showing an overall response rate of 65% in PI refractory patients [112, 113]. Importantly, the regimen was very well tolerated and did not have significant toxicity in addition to the expected toxicity of bortezomib. The integrated stress response (ISR) is a cellular stress response pathway activated in order to restore homeostasis in response to a number of stressors, including ER-stress. The ISR includes the UPR, and ultimately results in activation of ATF4, CHOP, and NOXA, but is also able to be activated outside of the context of ER-stress. Lymphoma and MM cells are sensitive to the UPR, and many mechanisms of resistance to PIs are the result of cellular changes to prevent PIs from causing ER-stress and induction of the UPR (e.g., plasmacytic differentiation, increased proteasome synthesis). As such, activation of the ISR by a mechanism not involving the UPR is a potential pathway to overcome PI resistance. A novel class of drugs, imipridones, is able to independently activate the ISR. ONC201, the first member of this class of drugs, is a dopamine receptor D-2 (DRD2) antagonist that activates the ISR without inducing ER-stress. Inhibition of DRD2 results in activation of EIF2α kinase 4 (GCN2), which activates ATF4, and induces apoptosis through CHOP and NOXA [114, 115]. Preclinical studies have shown activity in MM and early clinical phase studies are underway [116–118].

BCL-2 Inhibition

The final pathway of PIs is induction of apoptosis by expression of NOXA, which binds to MCL-1 leading to the release of BAK. Alterations in the expression of BCL-2 proteins can affect the sensitivity to PIs [119]. In a study of global DNA methylation in MCL, treatment with bortezomib resulted in hypomethylation across many *BCL* genes, in particular *NOXA*. It is not clear if alterations in this methylation pattern are responsible for PI resistance; however, the hypomethylating agent decitabine was able to induce further hypomethylation and synergizes with bortezomib in vitro and in a mouse model [120]. These results were confirmed by a separate group in MM cell lines [121]. Coadministration of bortezomib, to inhibit MCL-1, and venetoclax, to inhibit BCL-2, act synergistically and are able to overcome bortezomib resistance in lymphoma and MM cell lines [122–124]. In MM, venetoclax has been studied both as monotherapy and in combination with bortezomib. In heavily pretreated patients, monotherapy with venetoclax had very modest activity, but there were significantly more responses seen in patients with t(4;14), which correlates with BCL-2 expression [125]. In contrast, combined inhibition of MCL-1 and BCL-2 with bortezomib and venetoclax in a heavily pretreated population resulted in an overall response rate of 67% including a response rate of 24% in patients refractory to bortezomib [126].

Conclusion

The development of resistance to PIs in lymphoma is a complex process with multiple mechanisms. The most important mechanisms of resistance relate to an imbalance of proteasome demand and capacity which can be due to plasmacytic differentiation with its many causes, TJP1 and proteasome subunit production, and alternative protein degradation pathways such as autophagy. While the end result of each of these pathways is changes to how the cell responds to ER stress, the independent mechanisms offer multiple therapeutic options to overcome resistance. However, with multiple mechanisms of resistance, it is important to recognize that not all mechanisms of resistance will be clinically meaningful in all patients. As clinical trials are developed to overcome resistance, it will be important to include testing to evaluate the mechanisms of resistance implicated in individual patients with the goal in the future to identifying predictive biomarkers that can guide therapeutic decisions.

Conflicts of Interest No potential conflicts of interest were disclosed.

References

1. Robak T, Huang H, Jin J, Zhu J, Liu T, Samoilova O, Pylypenko H, Verhoef G, Siritanaratkul N, Osmanov E, Alexeeva J, Pereira J, Drach J, Mayer J, Hong X, Okamoto R, Pei L, Rooney B, van de Velde H, Cavalli F. Bortezomib-based therapy for newly diagnosed mantle-cell lymphoma. N Engl J Med. 2015;372:944–53.
2. Coiffier B, Osmanov EA, Hong X, Scheliga A, Mayer J, Offner F, Rule S, Teixeira A, Walewski J, de Vos S, Crump M, Shpilberg O, Esseltine DL, Zhu E, Enny C, Theocharous P, van de Velde H, Elsayed YA, Zinzani PL. Bortezomib plus rituximab versus rituximab alone in patients with relapsed, rituximab-naive or rituximab-sensitive, follicular lymphoma: a randomised phase 3 trial. Lancet Oncol. 2011;12:773–84.
3. Offner F, Samoilova O, Osmanov E, Eom HS, Topp MS, Raposo J, Pavlov V, Ricci D, Chaturvedi S, Zhu E, van de Velde H, Enny C, Rizo A, Ferhanoglu B. Frontline rituximab, cyclophosphamide, doxorubicin, and prednisone with bortezomib (VR-CAP) or vincristine (R-CHOP) for non-GCB DLBCL. Blood. 2015;126:1893–901.
4. Treon SP, Ioakimidis L, Soumerai JD, Patterson CJ, Sheehy P, Nelson M, Willen M, Matous J, Mattern J, Diener JG, Keogh GP, Myers TJ, Boral A, Birner A, Esseltine DL, Ghobrial IM. Primary therapy of Waldenstrom macroglobulinemia with bortezomib, dexamethasone, and rituximab: WMCTG clinical trial 05-180. J Clin Oncol. 2009;27:3830–5.
5. Sahasrabuddhe AA, Elenitoba-Johnson KS. Role of the ubiquitin proteasome system in hematologic malignancies. Immunol Rev. 2015;263:224–39.
6. Livneh I, Cohen-Kaplan V, Cohen-Rosenzweig C, Avni N, Ciechanover A. The life cycle of the 26S proteasome: from birth, through regulation and function, and onto its death. Cell Res. 2016;26:869–85.
7. Kuhn DJ, Hunsucker SA, Chen Q, Voorhees PM, Orlowski M, Orlowski RZ. Targeted inhibition of the immunoproteasome is a potent strategy against models of multiple myeloma that overcomes resistance to conventional drugs and nonspecific proteasome inhibitors. Blood. 2009;113:4667–76.
8. LeBlanc R, Catley LP, Hideshima T, Lentzsch S, Mitsiades CS, Mitsiades N, Neuberg D, Goloubeva O, Pien CS, Adams J, Gupta D, Richardson PG, Munshi NC, Anderson KC. Proteasome inhibitor PS-341 inhibits human myeloma cell growth in vivo and prolongs survival in a murine model. Cancer Res. 2002;62:4996–5000.
9. Groll M, Berkers CR, Ploegh HL, Ovaa H. Crystal structure of the boronic acid-based proteasome inhibitor bortezomib in complex with the yeast 20S proteasome. Structure. 2006;14:451–6.
10. Demo SD, Kirk CJ, Aujay MA, Buchholz TJ, Dajee M, Ho MN, Jiang J, Laidig GJ, Lewis ER, Parlati F, Shenk KD, Smyth MS, Sun CM, Vallone MK, Woo TM, Molineaux CJ, Bennett MK. Antitumor activity of PR-171, a novel irreversible inhibitor of the proteasome. Cancer Res. 2007;67:6383–91.
11. Lee EC, Fitzgerald M, Bannerman B, Donelan J, Bano K, Terkelsen J, Bradley DP, Subakan O, Silva MD, Liu R, Pickard M, Li Z, Tayber O, Li P, Hales P, Carsillo M, Neppalli VT, Berger AJ, Kupperman E, Manfredi M, Bolen JB, Van Ness B, Janz S. Antitumor activity of

the investigational proteasome inhibitor MLN9708 in mouse models of B-cell and plasma cell malignancies. Clin Cancer Res. 2011;17:7313–23.
12. Hideshima T, Chauhan D, Richardson P, Mitsiades C, Mitsiades N, Hayashi T, Munshi N, Dang L, Castro A, Palombella V, Adams J, Anderson KC. NF-kappa B as a therapeutic target in multiple myeloma. J Biol Chem. 2002;277:16639–47.
13. Mulligan G, Mitsiades C, Bryant B, Zhan F, Chng WJ, Roels S, Koenig E, Fergus A, Huang Y, Richardson P, Trepicchio WL, Broyl A, Sonneveld P, Shaughnessy JD Jr, Bergsagel PL, Schenkein D, Esseltine DL, Boral A, Anderson KC. Gene expression profiling and correlation with outcome in clinical trials of the proteasome inhibitor bortezomib. Blood. 2007;109:3177–88.
14. Hideshima T, Ikeda H, Chauhan D, Okawa Y, Raje N, Podar K, Mitsiades C, Munshi NC, Richardson PG, Carrasco RD, Anderson KC. Bortezomib induces canonical nuclear factor-kappaB activation in multiple myeloma cells. Blood. 2009;114:1046–52.
15. Lee AH, Iwakoshi NN, Anderson KC, Glimcher LH. Proteasome inhibitors disrupt the unfolded protein response in myeloma cells. Proc Natl Acad Sci U S A. 2003;100:9946–51.
16. Rasche L, Menoret E, Dubljevic V, Menu E, Vanderkerken K, Lapa C, Steinbrunn T, Chatterjee M, Knop S, Dull J, Greenwood DL, Hensel F, Rosenwald A, Einsele H, Brandlein S. A GRP78-directed monoclonal antibody recaptures response in refractory multiple myeloma with extramedullary involvement. Clin Cancer Res. 2016;22:4341–9.
17. Lin JH, Li H, Yasumura D, Cohen HR, Zhang C, Panning B, Shokat KM, Lavail MM, Walter P. IRE1 signaling affects cell fate during the unfolded protein response. Science. 2007;318:944–9.
18. Walter F, Schmid J, Dussmann H, Concannon CG, Prehn JH. Imaging of single cell responses to ER stress indicates that the relative dynamics of IRE1/XBP1 and PERK/ATF4 signalling rather than a switch between signalling branches determine cell survival. Cell Death Differ. 2015;22:1502–16.
19. Perez-Galan P, Roue G, Villamor N, Montserrat E, Campo E, Colomer D. The proteasome inhibitor bortezomib induces apoptosis in mantle-cell lymphoma through generation of ROS and Noxa activation independent of p53 status. Blood. 2006;107:257–64.
20. Wang Q, Mora-Jensen H, Weniger MA, Perez-Galan P, Wolford C, Hai T, Ron D, Chen W, Trenkle W, Wiestner A, Ye Y. ERAD inhibitors integrate ER stress with an epigenetic mechanism to activate BH3-only protein NOXA in cancer cells. Proc Natl Acad Sci U S A. 2009;106:2200–5.
21. Shamas-Din A, Brahmbhatt H, Leber B, Andrews DW. BH3-only proteins: Orchestrators of apoptosis. Biochim Biophys Acta. 2011;1813:508–20.
22. Qin JZ, Ziffra J, Stennett L, Bodner B, Bonish BK, Chaturvedi V, Bennett F, Pollock PM, Trent JM, Hendrix MJ, Rizzo P, Miele L, Nickoloff BJ. Proteasome inhibitors trigger NOXA-mediated apoptosis in melanoma and myeloma cells. Cancer Res. 2005;65:6282–93.
23. Baou M, Kohlhaas SL, Butterworth M, Vogler M, Dinsdale D, Walewska R, Majid A, Eldering E, Dyer MJ, Cohen GM. Role of NOXA and its ubiquitination in proteasome inhibitor-induced apoptosis in chronic lymphocytic leukemia cells. Haematologica. 2010;95:1510–8.
24. Nikiforov MA, Riblett M, Tang WH, Gratchouck V, Zhuang D, Fernandez Y, Verhaegen M, Varambally S, Chinnaiyan AM, Jakubowiak AJ, Soengas MS. Tumor cell-selective regulation of NOXA by c-MYC in response to proteasome inhibition. Proc Natl Acad Sci USA. 2007;104:19488–93.
25. Jullig M, Zhang WV, Ferreira A, Stott NS. MG132 induced apoptosis is associated with p53-independent induction of pro-apoptotic Noxa and transcriptional activity of beta-catenin. Apoptosis. 2006;11:627–41.
26. Olejniczak SH, Blickwedehl J, Belicha-Villanueva A, Bangia N, Riaz W, Mavis C, Clements JL, Gibbs J, Hernandez-Ilizaliturri FJ, Czuczman MS. Distinct molecular mechanisms responsible for bortezomib-induced death of therapy-resistant versus -sensitive B-NHL cells. Blood. 2010;116:5605–14.

27. Cillessen SA, Hijmering NJ, Moesbergen LM, Vos W, Verbrugge SE, Jansen G, Visser OJ, Oudejans JJ, Meijer CJ. ALK-negative anaplastic large cell lymphoma is sensitive to bortezomib through Noxa upregulation and release of Bax from Bcl-2. Haematologica. 2015;100:e365–8.
28. Dong H, Chen L, Chen X, Gu H, Gao G, Gao Y, Dong B. Dysregulation of unfolded protein response partially underlies proapoptotic activity of bortezomib in multiple myeloma cells. Leuk Lymphoma. 2009;50:974–84.
29. Hu J, Dang N, Menu E, De Bruyne E, Xu D, Van Camp B, Van Valckenborgh E, Vanderkerken K. Activation of ATF4 mediates unwanted Mcl-1 accumulation by proteasome inhibition. Blood. 2012;119:826–37.
30. Lu S, Yang J, Song X, Gong S, Zhou H, Guo L, Song N, Bao X, Chen P, Wang J. Point mutation of the proteasome beta5 subunit gene is an important mechanism of bortezomib resistance in bortezomib-selected variants of Jurkat T cell lymphoblastic lymphoma/leukemia line. J Pharmacol Exp Ther. 2008;326:423–31.
31. Ri M, Iida S, Nakashima T, Miyazaki H, Mori F, Ito A, Inagaki A, Kusumoto S, Ishida T, Komatsu H, Shiotsu Y, Ueda R. Bortezomib-resistant myeloma cell lines: a role for mutated PSMB5 in preventing the accumulation of unfolded proteins and fatal ER stress. Leukemia. 2010;24:1506–12.
32. Verbrugge SE, Assaraf YG, Dijkmans BA, Scheffer GL, Al M, den Uyl D, Oerlemans R, Chan ET, Kirk CJ, Peters GJ, van der Heijden JW, de Gruijl TD, Scheper RJ, Jansen G. Inactivating PSMB5 mutations and P-glycoprotein (multidrug resistance-associated protein/ATP-binding cassette B1) mediate resistance to proteasome inhibitors: ex vivo efficacy of (immuno) proteasome inhibitors in mononuclear blood cells from patients with rheumatoid arthritis. J Pharmacol Exp Ther. 2012;341:174–82.
33. Franke NE, Niewerth D, Assaraf YG, van Meerloo J, Vojtekova K, van Zantwijk CH, Zweegman S, Chan ET, Kirk CJ, Geerke DP, Schimmer AD, Kaspers GJ, Jansen G, Cloos J. Impaired bortezomib binding to mutant beta5 subunit of the proteasome is the underlying basis for bortezomib resistance in leukemia cells. Leukemia. 2012;26:757–68.
34. Oerlemans R, Franke NE, Assaraf YG, Cloos J, van Zantwijk I, Berkers CR, Scheffer GL, Debipersad K, Vojtekova K, Lemos C, van der Heijden JW, Ylstra B, Peters GJ, Kaspers GL, Dijkmans BA, Scheper RJ, Jansen G. Molecular basis of bortezomib resistance: proteasome subunit beta5 (PSMB5) gene mutation and overexpression of PSMB5 protein. Blood. 2008;112:2489–99.
35. Lu S, Yang J, Chen Z, Gong S, Zhou H, Xu X, Wang J. Different mutants of PSMB5 confer varying bortezomib resistance in T lymphoblastic lymphoma/leukemia cells derived from the Jurkat cell line. Exp Hematol. 2009;37:831–7.
36. Chapman MA, Lawrence MS, Keats JJ, Cibulskis K, Sougnez C, Schinzel AC, Harview CL, Brunet JP, Ahmann GJ, Adli M, Anderson KC, Ardlie KG, Auclair D, Baker A, Bergsagel PL, Bernstein BE, Drier Y, Fonseca R, Gabriel SB, Hofmeister CC, Jagannath S, Jakubowiak AJ, Krishnan A, Levy J, Liefeld T, Lonial S, Mahan S, Mfuko B, Monti S, Perkins LM, Onofrio R, Pugh TJ, Rajkumar SV, Ramos AH, Siegel DS, Sivachenko A, Stewart AK, Trudel S, Vij R, Voet D, Winckler W, Zimmerman T, Carpten J, Trent J, Hahn WC, Garraway LA, Meyerson M, Lander ES, Getz G, Golub TR. Initial genome sequencing and analysis of multiple myeloma. Nature. 2011;471:467–72.
37. Lichter DI, Danaee H, Pickard MD, Tayber O, Sintchak M, Shi H, Richardson PG, Cavenagh J, Blade J, Facon T, Niesvizky R, Alsina M, Dalton W, Sonneveld P, Lonial S, van de Velde H, Ricci D, Esseltine DL, Trepicchio WL, Mulligan G, Anderson KC. Sequence analysis of beta-subunit genes of the 20S proteasome in patients with relapsed multiple myeloma treated with bortezomib or dexamethasone. Blood. 2012;120:4513–6.
38. Politou M, Karadimitris A, Terpos E, Kotsianidis I, Apperley JF, Rahemtulla A. No evidence of mutations of the PSMB5 (beta-5 subunit of proteasome) in a case of myeloma with clinical resistance to Bortezomib. Leuk Res. 2006;30:240–1.

39. Wang L, Kumar S, Fridley BL, Kalari KR, Moon I, Pelleymounter LL, Hildebrandt MA, Batzler A, Eckloff BW, Wieben ED, Greipp PR. Proteasome beta subunit pharmacogenomics: gene resequencing and functional genomics. Clin Cancer Res. 2008;14:3503–13.
40. Fletcher JI, Haber M, Henderson MJ, Norris MD. ABC transporters in cancer: more than just drug efflux pumps. Nat Rev Cancer. 2010;10:147–56.
41. Katayama K, Noguchi K, Sugimoto Y. FBXO15 regulates P-glycoprotein/ABCB1 expression through the ubiquitin--proteasome pathway in cancer cells. Cancer Sci. 2013;104:694–702.
42. Minderman H, Zhou Y, O'Loughlin KL, Baer MR. Bortezomib activity and in vitro interactions with anthracyclines and cytarabine in acute myeloid leukemia cells are independent of multidrug resistance mechanisms and p53 status. Cancer Chemother Pharmacol. 2007;60:245–55.
43. Clemens J, Seckinger A, Hose D, Theile D, Longo M, Haefeli WE, Burhenne J, Weiss J. Cellular uptake kinetics of bortezomib in relation to efficacy in myeloma cells and the influence of drug transporters. Cancer Chemother Pharmacol. 2015;75:281–91.
44. Milan E, Fabbri M, Cenci S. Autophagy in plasma cell ontogeny and malignancy. J Clin Immunol. 2016;36(Suppl 1):18–24.
45. Ding WX, Ni HM, Gao W, Yoshimori T, Stolz DB, Ron D, Yin XM. Linking of autophagy to ubiquitin-proteasome system is important for the regulation of endoplasmic reticulum stress and cell viability. Am J Pathol. 2007;171:513–24.
46. Milani M, Rzymski T, Mellor HR, Pike L, Bottini A, Generali D, Harris AL. The role of ATF4 stabilization and autophagy in resistance of breast cancer cells treated with Bortezomib. Cancer Res. 2009;69:4415–23.
47. Zang Y, Thomas SM, Chan ET, Kirk CJ, Freilino ML, DeLancey HM, Grandis JR, Li C, Johnson DE. Carfilzomib and ONX 0912 inhibit cell survival and tumor growth of head and neck cancer and their activities are enhanced by suppression of Mcl-1 or autophagy. Clin Cancer Res. 2012;18:5639–49.
48. Jia L, Gopinathan G, Sukumar JT, Gribben JG. Blocking autophagy prevents bortezomib-induced NF-kappaB activation by reducing I-kappaBalpha degradation in lymphoma cells. PLoS One. 2012;7:e32584.
49. Hideshima T, Bradner JE, Wong J, Chauhan D, Richardson P, Schreiber SL, Anderson KC. Small-molecule inhibition of proteasome and aggresome function induces synergistic antitumor activity in multiple myeloma. Proc Natl Acad Sci USA. 2005;102:8567–72.
50. San-Miguel JF, Hungria VT, Yoon SS, Beksac M, Dimopoulos MA, Elghandour A, Jedrzejczak WW, Gunther A, Nakorn TN, Siritanaratkul N, Corradini P, Chuncharunee S, Lee JJ, Schlossman RL, Shelekhova T, Yong K, Tan D, Numbenjapon T, Cavenagh JD, Hou J, LeBlanc R, Nahi H, Qiu L, Salwender H, Pulini S, Moreau P, Warzocha K, White D, Blade J, Chen W, de la Rubia J, Gimsing P, Lonial S, Kaufman JL, Ocio EM, Veskovski L, Sohn SK, Wang MC, Lee JH, Einsele H, Sopala M, Corrado C, Bengoudifa BR, Binlich F, Richardson PG. Panobinostat plus bortezomib and dexamethasone versus placebo plus bortezomib and dexamethasone in patients with relapsed or relapsed and refractory multiple myeloma: a multicentre, randomised, double-blind phase 3 trial. Lancet Oncol. 2014;15:1195–206.
51. Amengual JE, Johannet P, Lombardo M, Zullo K, Hoehn D, Bhagat G, Scotto L, Jirau-Serrano X, Radeski D, Heinen J, Jiang H, Cremers S, Zhang Y, Jones S, O'Connor OA. Dual targeting of protein degradation pathways with the selective HDAC6 inhibitor ACY-1215 and Bortezomib is synergistic in lymphoma. Clin Cancer Res. 2015;21:4663–75.
52. Reimold AM, Iwakoshi NN, Manis J, Vallabhajosyula P, Szomolanyi-Tsuda E, Gravallese EM, Friend D, Grusby MJ, Alt F, Glimcher LH. Plasma cell differentiation requires the transcription factor XBP-1. Nature. 2001;412:300–7.
53. Iwakoshi NN, Lee AH, Vallabhajosyula P, Otipoby KL, Rajewsky K, Glimcher LH. Plasma cell differentiation and the unfolded protein response intersect at the transcription factor XBP-1. Nat Immunol. 2003;4:321–9.
54. Perez-Galan P, Mora-Jensen H, Weniger MA, Shaffer AL, Rizzatti EG, Chapman CM, Mo CC, Stennett LS, Rader C, Liu P, Raghavachari N, Stetler-Stevenson M, Yuan C, Pittaluga S,

Maric I, Dunleavy KM, Wilson WH, Staudt LM, Wiestner A. Bortezomib resistance in mantle cell lymphoma is associated with plasmacytic differentiation. Blood. 2011;117:542–52.
55. Kronke J, Udeshi ND, Narla A, Grauman P, Hurst SN, McConkey M, Svinkina T, Heckl D, Comer E, Li X, Ciarlo C, Hartman E, Munshi N, Schenone M, Schreiber SL, Carr SA, Ebert BL. Lenalidomide causes selective degradation of IKZF1 and IKZF3 in multiple myeloma cells. Science. 2014;343:301–5.
56. Lu G, Middleton RE, Sun H, Naniong M, Ott CJ, Mitsiades CS, Wong KK, Bradner JE, Kaelin WG Jr. The myeloma drug lenalidomide promotes the cereblon-dependent destruction of Ikaros proteins. Science. 2014;343:305–9.
57. Meister S, Schubert U, Neubert K, Herrmann K, Burger R, Gramatzki M, Hahn S, Schreiber S, Wilhelm S, Herrmann M, Jack HM, Voll RE. Extensive immunoglobulin production sensitizes myeloma cells for proteasome inhibition. Cancer Res. 2007;67:1783–92.
58. Gu JL, Li J, Zhou ZH, Liu JR, Huang BH, Zheng D, Su C. Differentiation induction enhances bortezomib efficacy and overcomes drug resistance in multiple myeloma. Biochem Biophys Res Commun. 2012;420:644–50.
59. Bianchi G, Oliva L, Cascio P, Pengo N, Fontana F, Cerruti F, Orsi A, Pasqualetto E, Mezghrani A, Calbi V, Palladini G, Giuliani N, Anderson KC, Sitia R, Cenci S. The proteasome load versus capacity balance determines apoptotic sensitivity of multiple myeloma cells to proteasome inhibition. Blood. 2009;113:3040–9.
60. Leung-Hagesteijn C, Erdmann N, Cheung G, Keats JJ, Stewart AK, Reece DE, Chung KC, Tiedemann RE. Xbp1s-negative tumor B cells and pre-plasmablasts mediate therapeutic proteasome inhibitor resistance in multiple myeloma. Cancer Cell. 2013;24:289–304.
61. Xu X, Liu J, Huang B, Chen M, Yuan S, Li X, Li J. Reduced response of IRE1alpha/Xbp-1 signaling pathway to bortezomib contributes to drug resistance in multiple myeloma cells. Tumori. 2016;103(3):261–7.
62. Ling SC, Lau EK, Al-Shabeeb A, Nikolic A, Catalano A, Iland H, Horvath N, Ho PJ, Harrison S, Fleming S, Joshua DE, Allen JD. Response of myeloma to the proteasome inhibitor bortezomib is correlated with the unfolded protein response regulator XBP-1. Haematologica. 2012;97:64–72.
63. Zhang XD, Baladandayuthapani V, Lin H, Mulligan G, Li B, Esseltine DL, Qi L, Xu J, Hunziker W, Barlogie B, Usmani SZ, Zhang Q, Crowley J, Hoering A, Shah JJ, Weber DM, Manasanch EE, Thomas SK, Li BZ, Wang HH, Zhang J, Kuiatse I, Tang JL, Wang H, He J, Yang J, Milan E, Cenci S, Ma WC, Wang ZQ, Davis RE, Yang L, Orlowski RZ. Tight junction protein 1 modulates proteasome capacity and proteasome inhibitor sensitivity in multiple myeloma via EGFR/JAK1/STAT3 signaling. Cancer Cell. 2016;29:639–52.
64. Yao Y, Sun Y, Shi M, Xia D, Zhao K, Zeng L, Yao R, Zhang Y, Li Z, Niu M, Xu K. Piperlongumine induces apoptosis and reduces bortezomib resistance by inhibiting STAT3 in multiple myeloma cells. Oncotarget. 2016;7(45):73497.
65. Punnoose EA, Leverson JD, Peale F, Boghaert ER, Belmont LD, Tan N, Young A, Mitten M, Ingalla E, Darbonne WC, Oleksijew A, Tapang P, Yue P, Oeh J, Lee L, Maiga S, Fairbrother WJ, Amiot M, Souers AJ, Sampath D. Expression profile of BCL-2, BCL-XL, and MCL-1 predicts pharmacological response to the BCL-2 selective antagonist Venetoclax in multiple myeloma models. Mol Cancer Ther. 2016;15:1132–44.
66. Smith AJ, Dai H, Correia C, Takahashi R, Lee SH, Schmitz I, Kaufmann SH. Noxa/Bcl-2 protein interactions contribute to bortezomib resistance in human lymphoid cells. J Biol Chem. 2011;286:17682–92.
67. Kim J, Denu RA, Dollar BA, Escalante LE, Kuether JP, Callander NS, Asimakopoulos F, Hematti P. Macrophages and mesenchymal stromal cells support survival and proliferation of multiple myeloma cells. Br J Haematol. 2012;158:336–46.
68. Zheng Y, Cai Z, Wang S, Zhang X, Qian J, Hong S, Li H, Wang M, Yang J, Yi Q. Macrophages are an abundant component of myeloma microenvironment and protect myeloma cells from chemotherapy drug-induced apoptosis. Blood. 2009;114:3625–8.

69. Ribatti D, Vacca A. The role of monocytes-macrophages in vasculogenesis in multiple myeloma. Leukemia. 2009;23:1535–6.
70. Galletti G, Scielzo C, Barbaglio F, Rodriguez TV, Riba M, Lazarevic D, Cittaro D, Simonetti G, Ranghetti P, Scarfo L, Ponzoni M, Rocchi M, Corti A, Anselmo A, van Rooijen N, Klein C, Ries CH, Ghia P, De Palma M, Caligaris-Cappio F, Bertilaccio MT. Targeting macrophages sensitizes chronic lymphocytic leukemia to apoptosis and inhibits disease progression. Cell Rep. 2016;14:1748–60.
71. Garayoa M, Garcia JL, Santamaria C, Garcia-Gomez A, Blanco JF, Pandiella A, Hernandez JM, Sanchez-Guijo FM, del Canizo MC, Gutierrez NC, San Miguel JF. Mesenchymal stem cells from multiple myeloma patients display distinct genomic profile as compared with those from normal donors. Leukemia. 2009;23:1515–27.
72. Corre J, Mahtouk K, Attal M, Gadelorge M, Huynh A, Fleury-Cappellesso S, Danho C, Laharrague P, Klein B, Reme T, Bourin P. Bone marrow mesenchymal stem cells are abnormal in multiple myeloma. Leukemia. 2007;21:1079–88.
73. Arnulf B, Lecourt S, Soulier J, Ternaux B, Lacassagne MN, Crinquette A, Dessoly J, Sciaini AK, Benbunan M, Chomienne C, Fermand JP, Marolleau JP, Larghero J. Phenotypic and functional characterization of bone marrow mesenchymal stem cells derived from patients with multiple myeloma. Leukemia. 2007;21:158–63.
74. McNee G, Eales KL, Wei W, Williams DS, Barkhuizen A, Bartlett DB, Essex S, Anandram S, Filer A, Moss PA, Pratt G, Basu S, Davies CC, Tennant DA. Citrullination of histone H3 drives IL-6 production by bone marrow mesenchymal stem cells in MGUS and multiple myeloma. Leukemia. 2016;31(2):373–81.
75. Voorhees PM, Chen Q, Kuhn DJ, Small GW, Hunsucker SA, Strader JS, Corringham RE, Zaki MH, Nemeth JA, Orlowski RZ. Inhibition of interleukin-6 signaling with CNTO 328 enhances the activity of bortezomib in preclinical models of multiple myeloma. Clin Cancer Res. 2007;13:6469–78.
76. Ishikawa H, Tsuyama N, Kawano MM. Interleukin-6-induced proliferation of human myeloma cells associated with CD45 molecules. Int J Hematol. 2003;78:95–105.
77. Kolosenko I, Grander D, Tamm KP. IL-6 activated JAK/STAT3 pathway and sensitivity to Hsp90 inhibitors in multiple myeloma. Curr Med Chem. 2014;21:3042–7.
78. Lin H, Kolosenko I, Bjorklund AC, Protsyuk D, Osterborg A, Grander D, Tamm KP. An activated JAK/STAT3 pathway and CD45 expression are associated with sensitivity to Hsp90 inhibitors in multiple myeloma. Exp Cell Res. 2013;319:600–11.
79. Patz M, Pallasch CP, Wendtner CM. Critical role of microRNAs in chronic lymphocytic leukemia: overexpression of the oncogene PLAG1 by deregulated miRNAs. Leuk Lymphoma. 2010;51:1379–81.
80. Hao M, Zhang L, An G, Meng H, Han Y, Xie Z, Xu Y, Li C, Yu Z, Chang H, Qiu L. Bone marrow stromal cells protect myeloma cells from bortezomib induced apoptosis by suppressing microRNA-15a expression. Leuk Lymphoma. 2011;52:1787–94.
81. Li Y, Zhang B, Li W, Wang L, Yan Z, Li H, Yao Y, Yao R, Xu K, Li Z. MiR-15a/16 regulates the growth of myeloma cells, angiogenesis and antitumor immunity by inhibiting Bcl-2, VEGF-A and IL-17 expression in multiple myeloma. Leuk Res. 2016;49:73–9.
82. Loffler D, Brocke-Heidrich K, Pfeifer G, Stocsits C, Hackermuller J, Kretzschmar AK, Burger R, Gramatzki M, Blumert C, Bauer K, Cvijic H, Ullmann AK, Stadler PF, Horn F. Interleukin-6 dependent survival of multiple myeloma cells involves the Stat3-mediated induction of microRNA-21 through a highly conserved enhancer. Blood. 2007;110:1330–3.
83. Wang X, Li C, Ju S, Wang Y, Wang H, Zhong R. Myeloma cell adhesion to bone marrow stromal cells confers drug resistance by microRNA-21 up-regulation. Leuk Lymphoma. 2011;52:1991–8.
84. Leone E, Morelli E, Di Martino MT, Amodio N, Foresta U, Gulla A, Rossi M, Neri A, Giordano A, Munshi NC, Anderson KC, Tagliaferri P, Tassone P. Targeting miR-21 inhibits in vitro and in vivo multiple myeloma cell growth. Clin Cancer Res. 2013;19:2096–106.

85. Wang J, Hendrix A, Hernot S, Lemaire M, De Bruyne E, Van Valckenborgh E, Lahoutte T, De Wever O, Vanderkerken K, Menu E. Bone marrow stromal cell-derived exosomes as communicators in drug resistance in multiple myeloma cells. Blood. 2014;124:555–66.
86. Zhang L, Yang J, Qian J, Li H, Romaguera JE, Kwak LW, Wang M, Yi Q. Role of the microenvironment in mantle cell lymphoma: IL-6 is an important survival factor for the tumor cells. Blood. 2012;120:3783–92.
87. Blotta S, Jakubikova J, Calimeri T, Roccaro AM, Amodio N, Azab AK, Foresta U, Mitsiades CS, Rossi M, Todoerti K, Molica S, Morabito F, Neri A, Tagliaferri P, Tassone P, Anderson KC, Munshi NC. Canonical and noncanonical Hedgehog pathway in the pathogenesis of multiple myeloma. Blood. 2012;120:5002–13.
88. Alonso S, Hernandez D, Chang YT, Gocke CD, McCray M, Varadhan R, Matsui WH, Jones RJ, Ghiaur G. Hedgehog and retinoid signaling alters multiple myeloma microenvironment and generates bortezomib resistance. J Clin Invest. 2016;126:4460–8.
89. Moros A, Rodriguez V, Saborit-Villarroya I, Montraveta A, Balsas P, Sandy P, Martinez A, Wiestner A, Normant E, Campo E, Perez-Galan P, Colomer D, Roue G. Synergistic antitumor activity of lenalidomide with the BET bromodomain inhibitor CPI203 in bortezomib-resistant mantle cell lymphoma. Leukemia. 2014;28:2049–59.
90. Mehta S, Singh C, Plata KB, Chanda PK, Paul A, Riosa S, Rosato RR, Rosato AE. Beta-Lactams increase the antibacterial activity of daptomycin against clinical methicillin-resistant Staphylococcus aureus strains and prevent selection of daptomycin-resistant derivatives. Antimicrob Agents Chemother. 2012;56:6192–200.
91. Voorhees PM, Manges RF, Sonneveld P, Jagannath S, Somlo G, Krishnan A, Lentzsch S, Frank RC, Zweegman S, Wijermans PW, Orlowski RZ, Kranenburg B, Hall B, Casneuf T, Qin X, van de Velde H, Xie H, Thomas SK. A phase 2 multicentre study of siltuximab, an anti-interleukin-6 monoclonal antibody, in patients with relapsed or refractory multiple myeloma. Br J Haematol. 2013;161:357–66.
92. Suzuki K, Ogura M, Abe Y, Suzuki T, Tobinai K, Ando K, Taniwaki M, Maruyama D, Kojima M, Kuroda J, Achira M, Iizuka K. Phase 1 study in Japan of siltuximab, an anti-IL-6 monoclonal antibody, in relapsed/refractory multiple myeloma. Int J Hematol. 2015;101:286–94.
93. Orlowski RZ, Gercheva L, Williams C, Sutherland H, Robak T, Masszi T, Goranova-Marinova V, Dimopoulos MA, Cavenagh JD, Spicka I, Maiolino A, Suvorov A, Blade J, Samoylova O, Puchalski TA, Reddy M, Bandekar R, van de Velde H, Xie H, Rossi JF. A phase 2, randomized, double-blind, placebo-controlled study of siltuximab (anti-IL-6 mAb) and bortezomib versus bortezomib alone in patients with relapsed or refractory multiple myeloma. Am J Hematol. 2015;90:42–9.
94. San-Miguel J, Blade J, Shpilberg O, Grosicki S, Maloisel F, Min CK, Polo Zarzuela M, Robak T, Prasad SV, Tee Goh Y, Laubach J, Spencer A, Mateos MV, Palumbo A, Puchalski T, Reddy M, Uhlar C, Qin X, van de Velde H, Xie H, Orlowski RZ. Phase 2 randomized study of bortezomib-melphalan-prednisone with or without siltuximab (anti-IL-6) in multiple myeloma. Blood. 2014;123:4136–42.
95. Sekulic A, Migden MR, Oro AE, Dirix L, Lewis KD, Hainsworth JD, Solomon JA, Yoo S, Arron ST, Friedlander PA, Marmur E, Rudin CM, Chang AL, Low JA, Mackey HM, Yauch RL, Graham RA, Reddy JC, Hauschild A. Efficacy and safety of vismodegib in advanced basal-cell carcinoma. N Engl J Med. 2012;366:2171–9.
96. Beauchamp EM, Ringer L, Bulut G, Sajwan KP, Hall MD, Lee YC, Peaceman D, Ozdemirli M, Rodriguez O, Macdonald TJ, Albanese C, Toretsky JA, Uren A. Arsenic trioxide inhibits human cancer cell growth and tumor development in mice by blocking Hedgehog/GLI pathway. J Clin Invest. 2011;121:148–60.
97. Kim J, Lee JJ, Kim J, Gardner D, Beachy PA. Arsenic antagonizes the Hedgehog pathway by preventing ciliary accumulation and reducing stability of the Gli2 transcriptional effector. Proc Natl Acad Sci U S A. 2010;107:13432–7.

98. Sanaat Z, Rezazadeh M, Gharamaleki JV, Ziae JE, Esfahani A. Arsenic trioxide in patients with refractory multiple myeloma: a prospective, phase II, single-arm study. Acta Med Iran. 2011;49:504–8.
99. Berenson JR, Matous J, Swift RA, Mapes R, Morrison B, Yeh HS. A phase I/II study of arsenic trioxide/bortezomib/ascorbic acid combination therapy for the treatment of relapsed or refractory multiple myeloma. Clin Cancer Res. 2007;13:1762–8.
100. Held LA, Rizzieri D, Long GD, Gockerman JP, Diehl LF, de Castro CM, Moore JO, Horwitz ME, Chao NJ, Gasparetto C. A Phase I study of arsenic trioxide (Trisenox), ascorbic acid, and bortezomib (Velcade) combination therapy in patients with relapsed/refractory multiple myeloma. Cancer Investig. 2013;31:172–6.
101. Gomaa MS, Bridgens CE, Veal GJ, Redfern CP, Brancale A, Armstrong JL, Simons C. Synthesis and biological evaluation of 3-(1H-imidazol- and triazol-1-yl)-2,2-dimethyl-3-[4-(naphthalen-2-ylamino)phenyl]propyl derivatives as small molecule inhibitors of retinoic acid 4-hydroxylase (CYP26). J Med Chem. 2011;54:6803–11.
102. Tan D, Phipps C, Hwang WY, Tan SY, Yeap CH, Chan YH, Tay K, Lim ST, Lee YS, Kumar SG, Ng SC, Fadilah S, Kim WS, Goh YT. Panobinostat in combination with bortezomib in patients with relapsed or refractory peripheral T-cell lymphoma: an open-label, multicentre phase 2 trial. Lancet Haematol. 2015;2:e326–33.
103. Dasmahapatra G, Lembersky D, Kramer L, Fisher RI, Friedberg J, Dent P, Grant S. The pan-HDAC inhibitor vorinostat potentiates the activity of the proteasome inhibitor carfilzomib in human DLBCL cells in vitro and in vivo. Blood. 2010;115:4478–87.
104. Bhatt S, Ashlock BM, Toomey NL, Diaz LA, Mesri EA, Lossos IS, Ramos JC. Efficacious proteasome/HDAC inhibitor combination therapy for primary effusion lymphoma. J Clin Invest. 2013;123:2616–28.
105. Frys S, Simons Z, Hu Q, Barth MJ, Gu JJ, Mavis C, Skitzki J, Song L, Czuczman MS, Hernandez-Ilizaliturri FJ. Entinostat, a novel histone deacetylase inhibitor is active in B-cell lymphoma and enhances the anti-tumour activity of rituximab and chemotherapy agents. Br J Haematol. 2015;169:506–19.
106. Roue G, Perez-Galan P, Mozos A, Lopez-Guerra M, Xargay-Torrent S, Rosich L, Saborit-Villarroya I, Normant E, Campo E, Colomer D. The Hsp90 inhibitor IPI-504 overcomes bortezomib resistance in mantle cell lymphoma in vitro and in vivo by down-regulation of the prosurvival ER chaperone BiP/Grp78. Blood. 2011;117:1270–9.
107. Frassanito MA, De Veirman K, Desantis V, Di Marzo L, Vergara D, Ruggieri S, Annese T, Nico B, Menu E, Catacchio I, Ria R, Racanelli V, Maffia M, Angelucci E, Derudas D, Fumarulo R, Dammacco F, Ribatti D, Vanderkerken K, Vacca A. Halting pro-survival autophagy by TGFbeta inhibition in bone marrow fibroblasts overcomes bortezomib resistance in multiple myeloma patients. Leukemia. 2016;30:640–8.
108. Guan M, Fousek K, Jiang C, Guo S, Synold T, Xi B, Shih CC, Chow WA. Nelfinavir induces liposarcoma apoptosis through inhibition of regulated intramembrane proteolysis of SREBP-1 and ATF6. Clin Cancer Res. 2011;17:1796–806.
109. Bono C, Karlin L, Harel S, Mouly E, Labaume S, Galicier L, Apcher S, Sauvageon H, Fermand JP, Bories JC, Arnulf B. The human immunodeficiency virus-1 protease inhibitor nelfinavir impairs proteasome activity and inhibits the proliferation of multiple myeloma cells in vitro and in vivo. Haematologica. 2012;97:1101–9.
110. Pyrko P, Kardosh A, Wang W, Xiong W, Schonthal AH, Chen TC. HIV-1 protease inhibitors nelfinavir and atazanavir induce malignant glioma death by triggering endoplasmic reticulum stress. Cancer Res. 2007;67:10920–8.
111. Bruning A, Burger P, Vogel M, Rahmeh M, Gingelmaiers A, Friese K, Lenhard M, Burges A. Nelfinavir induces the unfolded protein response in ovarian cancer cells, resulting in ER vacuolization, cell cycle retardation and apoptosis. Cancer Biol Ther. 2009;8:226–32.
112. Driessen C, Kraus M, Joerger M, Rosing H, Bader J, Hitz F, Berset C, Xyrafas A, Hawle H, Berthod G, Overkleeft HS, Sessa C, Huitema A, Pabst T, von Moos R, Hess D, Mey UJ. Treatment with the HIV protease inhibitor nelfinavir triggers the unfolded protein response

and may overcome proteasome inhibitor resistance of multiple myeloma in combination with bortezomib: a phase I trial (SAKK 65/08). Haematologica. 2016;101:346–55.
113. Driessen C, Müller R, Novak U, Cantoni N, Betticher D, Mach N, Gregor M, Samaras P, Berset C, Rondeau S, Hawle H, Hitz F, Pabst T, Zander T. The HIV protease inhibitor nelfinavir in combination with Bortezomib and dexamethasone (NVd) has excellent activity in patients with advanced, proteasome inhibitor-refractory multiple myeloma: a multicenter phase II trial (SAKK 39/13). Blood. 2016;128:487.
114. Kline CL, Van den Heuvel AP, Allen JE, Prabhu VV, Dicker DT, El-Deiry WS. ONC201 kills solid tumor cells by triggering an integrated stress response dependent on ATF4 activation by specific eIF2alpha kinases. Sci Signal. 2016;9:ra18.
115. Ishizawa J, Kojima K, Chachad D, Ruvolo P, Ruvolo V, Jacamo RO, Borthakur G, Mu H, Zeng Z, Tabe Y, Allen JE, Wang Z, Ma W, Lee HC, Orlowski R, Sarbassov dos D, Lorenzi PL, Huang X, Neelapu SS, McDonnell T, Miranda RN, Wang M, Kantarjian H, Konopleva M, Davis RE, Andreeff M. ATF4 induction through an atypical integrated stress response to ONC201 triggers p53-independent apoptosis in hematological malignancies. Sci Signal. 2016;9:ra17.
116. Prabhu VV, Lulla A, Kline CL, Van den Heuvel PJ, Talekar MK, Wagner JM, Tarapore RS, Dicker DT, Garnett MJ, McDermott U, Benes CH, Pu JJ, Claxton DF, Oster W, Allen JE, El-Deiry WS. Single agent and combinatorial efficacy of first-in-class small molecule ONC201 in acute leukemia and multiple myeloma. Blood. 2016;128:2759.
117. Y-s T, He J, Liu H, Davis RE, Orlowski RZ, Allen JE, Yang J. ONC201 overcomes chemotherapy resistance by upregulation of Bim in multiple myeloma. Blood. 2016;128:4476.
118. Tu YS, He J, Liu H, Lee HC, Wang H, Ishizawa J, Allen JE, Andreeff M, Orlowski RZ, Davis RE, Yang J. The Imipridone ONC201 induces apoptosis and overcomes chemotherapy resistance by up-regulation of Bim in multiple myeloma. Neoplasia. 2017;19:772–80.
119. Touzeau C, Ryan J, Guerriero J, Moreau P, Chonghaile TN, Le Gouill S, Richardson P, Anderson K, Amiot M, Letai A. BH3 profiling identifies heterogeneous dependency on Bcl-2 family members in multiple myeloma and predicts sensitivity to BH3 mimetics. Leukemia. 2016;30:761–4.
120. Leshchenko VV, Kuo PY, Jiang Z, Weniger MA, Overbey J, Dunleavy K, Wilson WH, Wiestner A, Parekh S. Harnessing Noxa demethylation to overcome Bortezomib resistance in mantle cell lymphoma. Oncotarget. 2015;6:27332–42.
121. Cao Y, Qiu GQ, Wu HQ, Wang ZL, Lin Y, Wu W, Xie XB, Gu WY. Decitabine enhances bortezomib treatment in RPMI 8226 multiple myeloma cells. Mol Med Rep. 2016;14:3469–75.
122. Dousset C, Maiga S, Gomez-Bougie P, Le Coq J, Touzeau C, Moreau P, Le Gouill S, Chiron D, Pellat-Deceunynck C, Moreau-Aubry A, Amiot M. BH3 profiling as a tool to identify acquired resistance to venetoclax in multiple myeloma. Br J Haematol. 2016;179(4):684–8.
123. Touzeau C, Dousset C, Le Gouill S, Sampath D, Leverson JD, Souers AJ, Maiga S, Bene MC, Moreau P, Pellat-Deceunynck C, Amiot M. The Bcl-2 specific BH3 mimetic ABT-199: a promising targeted therapy for t(11;14) multiple myeloma. Leukemia. 2014;28:210–2.
124. Johnson-Farley N, Veliz J, Bhagavathi S, Bertino JR. ABT-199, a BH3 mimetic that specifically targets Bcl-2, enhances the antitumor activity of chemotherapy, bortezomib and JQ1 in "double hit" lymphoma cells. Leuk Lymphoma. 2015;56:2146–52.
125. Kumar S, Vij R, Kaufman JL, Mikhael J, Facon T, Pegourie B, Benboubker L, Gasparetto C, Amiot M, Moreau P, Alzate S, Ross J, Dunbar M, Xu T, Agarwal S, Leverson J, Maciag P, Verdugo M, Touzeau C. Venetoclax monotherapy for relapsed/refractory multiple myeloma: safety and efficacy results from a phase I study. Blood. 2016;128:488.
126. Moreau P, Chanan-Khan AA, Roberts AW, Agarwal AB, Facon T, Kumar S, Touzeau C, Cordero J, Ross J, Munasinghe W, Jia J, Salem AH, Leverson J, Maciag P, Verdugo M, Harrison SJ. Venetoclax combined with Bortezomib and dexamethasone for patients with relapsed/refractory multiple myeloma. Blood. 2016;128:975.

IMiD: Immunomodulatory Drug Lenalidomide (CC-5013; Revlimid) in the Treatment of Lymphoma: Insights into Clinical Use and Molecular Mechanisms

Pashtoon Murtaza Kasi and Grzegorsz S. Nowakowski

Abstract Immune modulation has been a focus of increasing interest particularly for patients with lymphoma through the new class of 'immunomodulatory drugs' called IMiDs. Lenalidomide is an oral thalidomide analogue drug that belongs to the second generation of IMiDs. The proposed mechanisms of action of lenalidomide and the IMiD class of drugs go beyond just traditional cytotoxicity. With further descriptions comes more knowledge of predictive markers as well as molecular mechanisms of resistance. These still are evolving areas of research. Furthermore, mechanisms of resistance to IMiDs and ways to overcome may be different in different tumor types. The goal of this chapter is to focus on the early descriptions and usage of the drug, and to the more recent understandings of mechanisms of resistance. The main focus is on lymphoma, particularly diffuse large B-cell lymphoma. Knowledge and molecular insights gained pertaining to potential methods of overcoming these methods of resistance from other tumor types are also presented.

Keywords Lenalidomide · IMiD · Lymphoma · Immunomodulatory · Revlimid · DLBCL · GCB · Non-GCB · Non-Hodgkin's Lymphoma

P. M. Kasi (✉)
Division of Oncology, College of Medicine and Oncology, Mayo Clinic,
Jacksonville, FL, USA
e-mail: kasi.pashtoon@mayo.edu

G. S. Nowakowski
Division of Hematology, Mayo Clinic, Rochester, MN, USA

Abbreviations

ABC	Activated B-cell subtype
ADCC	Antibody-dependent cellular cytotoxicity
COO	Cell of Origin
CTCAE	Common terminology criteria for adverse events
CtDNA	Circulating tumor DNA
DLBCL	Diffuse Large B-Cell Lymphoma
GCB	Germinal center B-cell-like type
IMiD	Immunomodulatory Drug
mAbs	Monoclonal antibodies
NHL	Non-Hodgkin's Lymphoma
Non-GCB	Non-germinal B-cell-like type
R2ICE	Combination chemoimmunotherapy regimen R-ICE with the addition of lenalidomide (Revlimid)
R-ICE	Combination chemoimmunotherapy regimen consisting of rituximab, ifosfamide, carboplatin and etoposide

Introduction

Non-Hodgkin's Lymphoma

Non-Hodgkin's lymphoma (NHL) is the most common type of lymphomas. Within NHL, diffuse large B-Cell lymphomas (DLBCL) are the most common. Therapies upfront for DLBCL include chemotherapeutic options in combination with biologics/monoclonal antibodies (mAbs), which are curative in intent. Even in the relapsed or refractory settings, the intent of the regimens for patients with DLBCL is to achieve cure; however, these have to be consolidated with a stem cell transplant (autologous in most instances). The number of treatment options is increasing and newer regimens and classes of drugs are being developed and tested for these patients. These go beyond mAbs and traditional chemotherapeutic agents, and include novel targeted therapies, immunotherapies and immunomodulatory agents. Immune modulation has been a focus of increasing interest particularly for patients with DBLCL through the new class of immunomodulatory drugs called IMiDs.

Lenalidomide for the Treatment of Lymphoma

Lenalidomide belongs to this new class of drugs referred to as IMiDs (immunomodulatory drugs). From its initial descriptions and few reports in early 2000s, the number of instances where lenalidomide and lymphoma are being described in the literature is increasing (Fig. 1) [1].

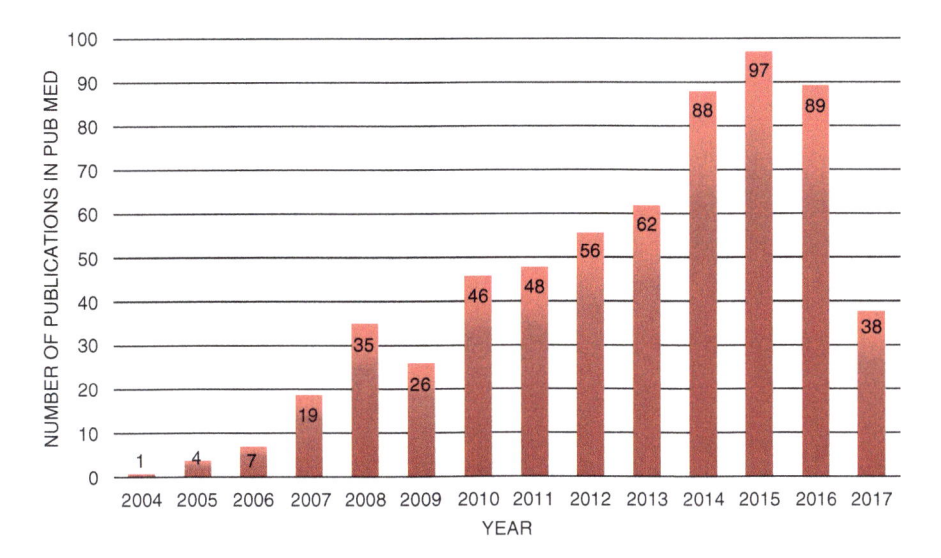

Fig. 1 Trend showing the increase in the number of publications with "lenalidomide" AND "lymphoma" from 2004 to 2017 to date

With further descriptions comes more knowledge of predictive markers as well as molecular mechanisms of resistance. The goal of this chapter is to focus on the early descriptions and usage of the drug and to the more recent understandings of mechanisms of resistance. We also propose and describe potential methods of overcoming these methods of resistance, and ways forward.

Of note, the drug lenalidomide is being used a variety of indications both as a single-agent and in combination with other drugs and immunotherapeutic agents. These include, for example, multiple myeloma and myelodysplastic syndrome (with deletion 5q) [2, 3]. The focus here would be on the use of lenalidomide in the treatment of lymphoma.

Structure and Mechanism of Action

Lenalidomide is a thalidomide analogue. Lenalidomide is an oral drug. As a single agent, dosing employed is typically once daily with maximum tolerated doses described up to 25 mg a day for 3 weeks on and 1 week off, depending on the previously reported clinical trials and indications studied.

The proposed mechanisms of action of lenalidomide and the IMiD class of drugs beyond just traditional cytotoxicity in general are shown in Fig. 2 [4].

From its parent compound, thalidomide's initial descriptions of its teratogenicity attributed to its anti-angiogenic properties, lenalidomide (CC-5013; Revlimid, Celgene®) has effects on multiple other aspects of the tumor and the tumor microenvironment. The drug belongs to the second generation of IMiDs. These are more potent and effective than their parent compound. In this particular chapter, we will

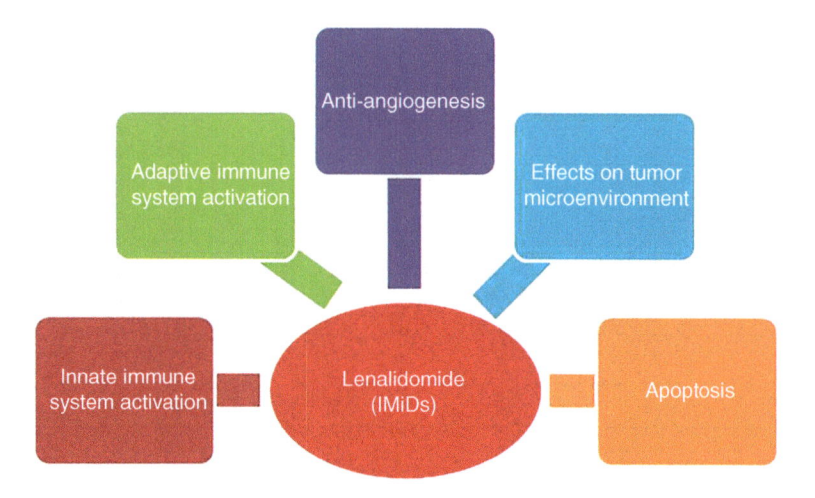

Fig. 2 Proposed mechanism of action of lenalidomide and the IMiD class of drugs beyond just traditional cytotoxicity

focus on the effects seen pertaining to the treatment of lymphoma. As shown in Fig. 2, the effects of lenalidomide include the activation of various aspects of the immune system of the host alongside effects on the tumor as well as the tumor microenvironment. From the host's perspective, it can affect both the innate as well as the adaptive immune systems (T-cell function). It appears to help the function of natural killer (NK) cells [5]. From a tumor microenvironment's perspective, it has anti-angiogenic properties and can also affect the milieu with many other downstream consequences through its effects on various cytokines e.g. tumor necrosis factor alpha (TNF-α), interferon-gamma (INF-γ) and other interleukins [6, 7]. Finally, it has direct effects on the lymphoma cell lines e.g. induction of apoptosis. "At the molecular level, lenalidomide cytotoxic activity relies on its binding to the E3-ligase adaptor cereblon (CRBN) selectively leading to CSNK1a protein degradation." [8]

Together with other drugs, its effects are further potentiated. For example, when used in conjunction with rituximab, lenalidomide appears to aid in one of the key mechanisms of actions of the mAb, which is antibody-dependent cellular cytotoxicity (ADCC) [9].

Toxicities

Even though lenalidomide is a more potent and an effective second generation IMiD, it has a different side effect profile as compared to its parent compound [2]. Beyond the traditional myelosuppressive effects (neutropenia, thrombocytopenia) seen with a lot of these and other compounds, the major source of concern when using lenalidomide is the incidence of thromboembolic events in these patients. Deep vein thrombosis can occur. This has prompted the use of low molecular weight heparin (LMWH),

Coumadin (warfarin) or at least an aspirin in patients who are not candidates for anticoagulation, depending on the indication and the combination in which lenalidomide is being tested. Arterial thrombotic events can also occur e.g. myocardial infarction or stroke; however, these are relatively infrequent as compared to venous thromboembolic events [10]. Patients at high risk of developing such events are not great candidates for the use of lenalidomide and are traditionally excluded from clinical trials using lenalidomide. This has prompted routine use of anticoagulation or at least antiplatelet agents as thromboprophylaxis for these patients [11].

Toxicities obviously are compounded and accentuated in instances of combination of the drug with other agents. As a single agent, common grade 3 adverse events (based on common terminology criteria for adverse events – CTCAE) are leucopenia, neutropenia and thrombocytopenia [12, 13]. A mild rash is commonly seen, but is manageable. In some trials, it was noted to be a predictive marker of response [14]. With multi-agent combination regimens, stem cell mobilization could potentially be affected and should be monitored on trials. With agents like plerixafor, mobilization is achieved even in instances of patients failing mobilization through traditional colony stimulating factors.

Other Insights from Preclinical Models

Several studies in predominantly lymphoma and myeloma cell lines and models have tried to explore further the mechanisms of action of lenalidomide and IMiDs. One study shows potential epigenetic mechanisms of action of lenalidomide in causing G_0-G_1 cell cycle arrest through increased expression of the $p21^{WAF-1}$ protein [15]. This has downstream consequences in cyclin-dependent kinase signaling. The authors show that these appear to be regulated through decreased methylation and increased histone acetylation; something not thought of before. Similar synergy and mechanism of action in terms of increasing dexamethasone induced G_0-G_1 cell cycle arrest were seen in mantle cell lymphoma cell lines and mouse models [16].

Clinical Indications and Data

With respect to patients with lymphoma, for many years the combination of rituximab to the CHOP regimen (cyclophosphamide, doxorubicin, vincristine and prednisone), R-CHOP regimen has remained the gold standard for patients with diffuse large B-cell lymphoma (DLBCL). The Hans classification further subdivides patients with DLBCL to germinal center B-cell-like type (GCB) and the non-germinal B-cell-like type (non-GCB). The latter non-GCB subtype is often referred to as the activated B-cell (ABC) subtype. It confers a poorer prognosis. Regimens trying to improve upon the efficacy of the R-CHOP have employed the addition of another agent to this combination. Various drugs (X) have been added and tested

(X + R-CHOP). These have had variable successes and increased toxicities. The addition of lenalidomide (R) to the R-CHOP, referred to as R2CHOP, significantly improved survival in patients with DLBCL [17]. In particular, patients with the non-GCB subtype who received the drug had a significant improvement in overall response rate and overall survival. This would be considered the new standard of care for patients with DLBCL with a large phase-3 trial currently exploring this question. This has also led to the addition of the lenalidomide (R) to the refractory regimens for patients with DLBCL; e.g. the addition of the drug to R-ICE (rituximab, ifosfamide, carboplatin and etoposide) regimen, to make the so-called R2ICE regimen. An ongoing phase-1/2 trial is currently accruing rapidly and has entered into the highest dose cohort level employing the traditional 3 + 3 design. The R2ICE trial is looking into improvement of overall response rates in patients with DLBCL (relapsed/refractory) after 2 cycles before eligible patients would proceed to an autologous stem cell transplant. Insights from such and other similar trials in the near future would further help personalize and stratify therapy for such patients. As a secondary outcome measure, it is important to note the number of patients able to achieve stem cell collection going for an autologous stem cell transplant given concerns regarding this being hampered in patients in the relapsed/refractory settings exposed to multiple prior lines of therapies.

The first reports of activity of using lenalidomide in patients with NHL came from studies using it as a single agent. A phase-2 clinical trial by Wiernek and colleagues reported an overall response rate (ORR) of 35% (12% complete response (CR)) [12]. The trial had a total of 49 patients who previously had received multiple lines of therapies. Most of these patients had DLBCL. Another study by Witzig et al. looking at this as single-agent in 43 patients with indolent NHL showed an ORR of 23% (7% CR) [18]. Similarly, an international trial incorporating 217 patients showed an ORR 35% (13% CR) [19]. The combination of lenalidomide with the mAb Rituximab showed an ORR of 35% in elderly patients with relapsed/refractory DLBCL [20]. Activity was also seen in a phase-2 clinical trial of patients with classical HL [21].

Predictive Markers for Lenalidomide in Patients with Lymphoma

In patients with DLBCL, the most common type of NHL, the most consistent predictive biomarker of response that has emerged is the presence of the non-GCB phenotype [22]. Now gene-expression profiling, which is readily becoming available, is also being incorporated in terms of differentiating between the two subtypes of DLBCL (GCB versus non-GCB). Cell of origin (COO) appears to be a marker in transformed lymphoma cases as well [23]. In these instances, lenalidomide at the molecular level appears to be acting through INF-β [24]. The presence of myeloid differentiation primary response 88 (MYD88) alterations in these tumors and the NF-κB pathway may be responsible for the effectiveness of lenalidomide in these situations.

Molecular Mechanisms of Resistance

Molecular mechanisms of resistance to novel agents are still an evolving area of research. Furthermore, mechanisms of resistance to IMiDs and ways to overcome may be different in different tumor types.

In patients with multiple myeloma, it might be related to changes in the expression of the target of IMiDs, the cereblon (CRBN) [25]. Gene expression profile was studied in these patients before and after treatment with lenalidomide. This shows complex up- as well as downregulation of different genes in different pathways. So the mechanism of resistance may not be as straightforward; and different subsets of patients in different studies are showing varied mechanisms. Bjorklund and colleagues were able to show that in plasma cell lines, this was mediated through the Wnt/β-Catenin pathway [26]. This, as proposed by the authors, could serve as a marker of sensitivity to the drug. Downstream activation of other proteins are also potential targets that could be exploited based on these findings. In a separate pre-clinical model of multiple myeloma xenograft models, resistance to IMiDs was mediated through the mitogen-activated protein kinase/extracellular signal-regulated kinase (ERK) kinase (MEK)/ERK pathway [27]. Interestingly, in this work by Ocio and colleagues looking at multiple aspects of drug resistance to both lenalidomide and the other IMiD pomalidomide, the resistance to both drugs was exclusive of one another. They showed in multiple experiments with cell lines being resistant to lenalidomide that were sensitive still to pomalidomide and vice versa, although the latter was less effective. Furthermore, exposure to a MEK-inhibitor could overcome this mechanism of resistance. Additionally, a washout period also accomplished the same, leading to potential implications of continuous exposure to the drug versus intermittent usage in the treatment of various malignancies [27]. In another study of multiple myeloma cell lines resistant to lenalidomide, the hepatocyte growth factor (HGF)/MET signaling pathway appeared to play a role, with the addition of crizotinib helping overcome this in preclinical models [28].

Similarly, in patients with multiple myeloma, clarithromycin when given in addition to lenalidomide and dexamethasone was able to overcome resistance in a fraction of patients who were noted to be resistant to the doublet [29]. The exact mechanism was thought to be related to not only the interaction of the drug with corticosteroids, but also potentially other immunomodulatory effects potentiating lenalidomide.

In contrast, in patients with Del (5q) myelodysplastic syndrome patients resistance was shown to be mediated through *TP53* mutations [8]. While some of these mutations conferred resistance if present at diagnosis, others were acquired and mediated resistance at progression of disease [8]. With circulating tumor DNA (ctDNA) based tests now increasingly and readily becoming available, further studies to look into these mechanisms of resistance e.g. acquired mutations would be easier to conduct.

Most of the work on molecular mechanisms of resistance as noted is done in patients with multiple myeloma and myelodysplastic syndrome where lenalidomide has been used for a longer period of time. Similar studies in patients with lymphoma incorporating tissue or liquid biopsies before and after treatment will help gain novel insights of mechanisms of resistance in this cohort of patients. Mechanisms of resistance may be different across tumor types. Furthermore, even within the same tumor types e.g. DLBCL, the degree of tumor heterogeneity that exists underscores further characterization of subsets of patients with potentially different mechanisms of resistance [30]. Finally, within the class of IMiDs, mechanisms of resistance may not be the same [31].

Future Directions

Lenalidomide alongside other IMiDs are being tested in various combinations with other drugs in both preclinical and clinical models. Several very intriguing observations have emerged. In a study by Verhelle and colleagues, the drug appears to have synergistic activity with the class of epigenetic drugs histone deacetylase (HDAC) inhibitors [32]. In the same study, lenalidomide was noted to have positive effects on the bone marrow by increasing the number of progenitor CD34+ cells.

Furthermore, there are an increasing number of malignancies where lenalidomide is showing promising activity. These include malignancies beyond NHL and myeloma, e.g. follicular lymphoma, mantle-cell lymphoma, T-Cell lymphomas, refractory acute leukemias, and other hematologic neoplasms [13, 14, 33–36]. In a clinical trial of 15 patients with mantle-cell lymphoma, lenalidomide as a single-agent achieved an ORR of 53% (20% CR) [13].

Clinical trials ongoing of note include the R2ICE for relapsed/refractory lymphoma and trials incorporating anti-programmed death-1 or programmed death-ligand-1 (PD1/PD-L1) receptor antibodies. The multitude of mechanisms through which it works beyond those described continues to be an area of ongoing research e.g. its effectiveness in MDS with 5q deletion [37].

The knowledge gained so far on the molecular mechanisms of resistance show diverse intra-class, inter-tumor as well as intra-tumor up- as well as down-regulation of key genes/pathways. The process appears to be dynamic and may not be applicable to all patients getting lenalidomide. Incorporation of targeted therapies e.g. MET or MEK inhibition in select patients exhibiting these changes appears to be a promising strategy. This further underscores the importance of reassessing the molecular profile of the tumor as it develops resistance to any of the novel therapies.

Conflict of Interest The authors declare no conflicts of interest.

References

1. Gibson AD, Klem J, Price N, Reddy GK. 45th annual meeting of the American Society of Hematology December 6–9, 2003. Clin Lymphoma. 2004;4(4):206–12.
2. Weber DM, Chen C, Niesvizky R, Wang M, Belch A, Stadtmauer EA, Siegel D, Borrello I, Rajkumar SV, Chanan-Khan AA, Lonial S, Yu Z, Patin J, Olesnyckyj M, Zeldis JB, Knight RD, Multiple Myeloma Study I. Lenalidomide plus dexamethasone for relapsed multiple myeloma in North America. N Engl J Med. 2007;357(21):2133–42.
3. Knop S, Einsele H, Bargou R, Cosgrove D, List A. Adjusted dose lenalidomide is safe and effective in patients with deletion (5q) myelodysplastic syndrome and severe renal impairment. Leuk Lymphoma. 2008;49(2):346–9.
4. Hernandez-Ilizaliturri FJ, Reddy N, Holkova B, Ottman E, Czuczman MS. Immunomodulatory drug CC-5013 or CC-4047 and rituximab enhance antitumor activity in a severe combined immunodeficient mouse lymphoma model. Clin Cancer Res. 2005;11(16):5984–92.
5. Zhu D, Corral LG, Fleming YW, Stein B. Immunomodulatory drugs Revlimid (lenalidomide) and CC-4047 induce apoptosis of both hematological and solid tumor cells through NK cell activation. Cancer Immunol Immunother. 2008;57(12):1849–59.
6. Crane E, List A. Immunomodulatory drugs. Cancer Investig. 2005;23(7):625–34.
7. Reddy N, Hernandez-Ilizaliturri FJ, Deeb G, Roth M, Vaughn M, Knight J, Wallace P, Czuczman MS. Immunomodulatory drugs stimulate natural killer-cell function, alter cytokine production by dendritic cells, and inhibit angiogenesis enhancing the anti-tumour activity of rituximab in vivo. Br J Haematol. 2008;140(1):36–45.
8. Martinez-Høyer S, Docking R, Chan S, Jadersten M, Parker J, Karsan A. Mechanisms of resistance to Lenalidomide in Del (5q) myelodysplastic syndrome patients. Blood. 2015;126(23):5228–5228.
9. Wu L, Adams M, Carter T, Chen R, Muller G, Stirling D, Schafer P, Bartlett JB. Lenalidomide enhances natural killer cell and monocyte-mediated antibody-dependent cellular cytotoxicity of rituximab-treated CD20+ tumor cells. Clin Cancer Res. 2008;14(14):4650–7.
10. Martin MG, Vij R. Arterial thrombosis with immunomodulatory derivatives in the treatment of multiple myeloma: a single-center case series and review of the literature. Clin Lymphoma Myeloma. 2009;9(4):320–3.
11. Niesvizky R, Martinez-Banos D, Jalbrzikowski J, Christos P, Furst J, De Sancho M, Mark T, Pearse R, Mazumdar M, Zafar F, Pekle K, Leonard J, Jayabalan D, Coleman M. Prophylactic low-dose aspirin is effective antithrombotic therapy for combination treatments of thalidomide or lenalidomide in myeloma. Leuk Lymphoma. 2007;48(12):2330–7.
12. Wiernik PH, Lossos IS, Tuscano JM, Justice G, Vose JM, Cole CE, Lam W, McBride K, Wride K, Pietronigro D, Takeshita K, Ervin-Haynes A, Zeldis JB, Habermann TM. Lenalidomide monotherapy in relapsed or refractory aggressive non-Hodgkin's lymphoma. J Clin Oncol. 2008;26(30):4952–7.
13. Habermann TM, Lossos IS, Justice G, Vose JM, Wiernik PH, McBride K, Wride K, Ervin-Haynes A, Takeshita K, Pietronigro D, Zeldis JB, Tuscano JM. Lenalidomide oral monotherapy produces a high response rate in patients with relapsed or refractory mantle cell lymphoma. Br J Haematol. 2009;145(3):344–9.
14. Dueck G, Chua N, Prasad A, Finch D, Stewart D, White D, van der Jagt R, Johnston J, Belch A, Reiman T. Interim report of a phase 2 clinical trial of lenalidomide for T-cell non-Hodgkin lymphoma. Cancer. 2010;116(19):4541–8.
15. Escoubet-Lozach L, Lin IL, Jensen-Pergakes K, Brady HA, Gandhi AK, Schafer PH, Muller GW, Worland PJ, Chan KW, Verhelle D. Pomalidomide and lenalidomide induce p21 WAF-1 expression in both lymphoma and multiple myeloma through a LSD1-mediated epigenetic mechanism. Cancer Res. 2009;69(18):7347–56.
16. Qian Z, Zhang L, Cai Z, Sun L, Wang H, Yi Q, Wang M. Lenalidomide synergizes with dexamethasone to induce growth arrest and apoptosis of mantle cell lymphoma cells in vitro and in vivo. Leuk Res. 2011;35(3):380–6.

17. Nowakowski GS, LaPlant B, Habermann TM, Rivera CE, Macon WR, Inwards DJ, Micallef IN, Johnston PB, Porrata LF, Ansell SM, Klebig RR, Reeder CB, Witzig TE. Lenalidomide can be safely combined with R-CHOP (R2CHOP) in the initial chemotherapy for aggressive B-cell lymphomas: phase I study. Leukemia. 2011;25(12):1877–81.
18. Witzig TE, Wiernik PH, Moore T, Reeder C, Cole C, Justice G, Kaplan H, Voralia M, Pietronigro D, Takeshita K, Ervin-Haynes A, Zeldis JB, Vose JM. Lenalidomide oral monotherapy produces durable responses in relapsed or refractory indolent non-Hodgkin's lymphoma. J Clin Oncol. 2009;27(32):5404–9.
19. Witzig TE, Vose JM, Zinzani PL, Reeder CB, Buckstein R, Polikoff JA, Bouabdallah R, Haioun C, Tilly H, Guo P, Pietronigro D, Ervin-Haynes AL, Czuczman MS. An international phase II trial of single-agent lenalidomide for relapsed or refractory aggressive B-cell non-Hodgkin's lymphoma. Ann Oncol. 2011;22(7):1622–7.
20. Zinzani PL, Pellegrini C, Gandolfi L, Stefoni V, Quirini F, Derenzini E, Broccoli A, Argnani L, Pileri S, Baccarani M. Combination of lenalidomide and rituximab in elderly patients with relapsed or refractory diffuse large B-cell lymphoma: a phase 2 trial. Clin Lymphoma Myeloma Leuk. 2011;11(6):462–6.
21. Fehniger TA, Larson S, Trinkaus K, Siegel MJ, Cashen AF, Blum KA, Fenske TS, Hurd DD, Goy A, Schneider SE, Keppel CR, Wagner-Johnston ND, Carson KR, Bartlett NL. A phase 2 multicenter study of lenalidomide in relapsed or refractory classical Hodgkin lymphoma. Blood. 2011;118(19):5119–25.
22. Hernandez-Ilizaliturri FJ, Deeb G, Zinzani PL, Pileri SA, Malik F, Macon WR, Goy A, Witzig TE, Czuczman MS. Higher response to lenalidomide in relapsed/refractory diffuse large B-cell lymphoma in nongerminal center B-cell-like than in germinal center B-cell-like phenotype. Cancer. 2011;117(22):5058–66.
23. Czuczman MS, Vose JM, Witzig TE, Zinzani PL, Buckstein R, Polikoff J, Li J, Pietronigro D, Ervin-Haynes A, Reeder CB. The differential effect of lenalidomide monotherapy in patients with relapsed or refractory transformed non-Hodgkin lymphoma of distinct histological origin. Br J Haematol. 2011;154(4):477–81.
24. Yang Y, Shaffer AL 3rd, Emre NC, Ceribelli M, Zhang M, Wright G, Xiao W, Powell J, Platig J, Kohlhammer H, Young RM, Zhao H, Yang Y, Xu W, Buggy JJ, Balasubramanian S, Mathews LA, Shinn P, Guha R, Ferrer M, Thomas C, Waldmann TA, Staudt LM. Exploiting synthetic lethality for the therapy of ABC diffuse large B cell lymphoma. Cancer Cell. 2012;21(6):723–37.
25. Amatangelo MD, Neri P, Ortiz M, Bjorklund CC, Gandhi AK, Klippel A, Bahlis NJ, Daniel T, Chopra R, Trotter M, Thakurta A. Resistance to Lenalidomide in multiple myeloma is associated with a switch in gene expression profile. Blood. 2015;126(23):1789–1789.
26. Bjorklund CC, Ma W, Wang ZQ, Davis RE, Kuhn DJ, Kornblau SM, Wang M, Shah JJ, Orlowski RZ. Evidence of a role for activation of Wnt/beta-catenin signaling in the resistance of plasma cells to lenalidomide. J Biol Chem. 2011;286(13):11009–20.
27. Ocio EM, Fernández-Lázaro D, San-Segundo L, Lopez-Corral L, Corchete LA, Gutiérrez NC, Garayoa M, Paíno T, García-Gómez A, Delgado M. In vivo murine model of acquired resistance in myeloma reveals differential mechanisms for lenalidomide and pomalidomide in combination with dexamethasone. Leukemia. 2015;29(3):705–14.
28. Zaman S, Stellrecht CM, Orlowski RZ, Gandhi V. Abstract 1710: Bortezomib and lenalidomide resistant myeloma cells overexpress the hepatocyte growth factor/MET signaling axis and respond to MET kinase inhibitors. Cancer Res. 2014;74(19 Supplement):1710.
29. Ghosh N, Tucker N, Zahurak M, Wozney J, Borrello I, Huff CA. Clarithromycin overcomes resistance to lenalidomide and dexamethasone in multiple myeloma. Am J Hematol. 2014;89(8):E116–20.
30. Turturro F. Constitutive NF-κB activation underlines major mechanism of drug resistance in relapsed refractory diffuse large B cell lymphoma. Biomed Res Int. 2015;2015:5.
31. Chanan-Khan AA, Swaika A, Paulus A, Kumar SK, Mikhael JR, Rajkumar SV, Dispenzieri A, Lacy MQ. Pomalidomide: the new immunomodulatory agent for the treatment of multiple myeloma. Blood Cancer J. 2013;3:e143.

32. Verhelle D, Corral LG, Wong K, Mueller JH, Moutouh-de Parseval L, Jensen-Pergakes K, Schafer PH, Chen R, Glezer E, Ferguson GD, Lopez-Girona A, Muller GW, Brady HA, Chan KW. Lenalidomide and CC-4047 inhibit the proliferation of malignant B cells while expanding normal CD34+ progenitor cells. Cancer Res. 2007;67(2):746–55.
33. Tempescul A, Ianotto JC, Morel F, Marion V, De Braekeleer M, Berthou C. Lenalidomide, as a single agent, induces complete remission in a refractory mantle cell lymphoma. Ann Hematol. 2009;88(9):921–2.
34. Ramsay AG, Clear AJ, Kelly G, Fatah R, Matthews J, Macdougall F, Lister TA, Lee AM, Calaminici M, Gribben JG. Follicular lymphoma cells induce T-cell immunologic synapse dysfunction that can be repaired with lenalidomide: implications for the tumor microenvironment and immunotherapy. Blood. 2009;114(21):4713–20.
35. Blum W, Klisovic RB, Becker H, Yang X, Rozewski DM, Phelps MA, Garzon R, Walker A, Chandler JC, Whitman SP, Curfman J, Liu S, Schaaf L, Mickle J, Kefauver C, Devine SM, Grever MR, Marcucci G, Byrd JC. Dose escalation of lenalidomide in relapsed or refractory acute leukemias. J Clin Oncol. 2010;28(33):4919–25.
36. Wang M, Fayad L, Wagner-Bartak N, Zhang L, Hagemeister F, Neelapu SS, Samaniego F, McLaughlin P, Fanale M, Younes A, Cabanillas F, Fowler N, Newberry KJ, Sun L, Young KH, Champlin R, Kwak L, Feng L, Badillo M, Bejarano M, Hartig K, Chen W, Chen Y, Byrne C, Bell N, Zeldis J, Romaguera J. Lenalidomide in combination with rituximab for patients with relapsed or refractory mantle-cell lymphoma: a phase 1/2 clinical trial. Lancet Oncol. 2012;13(7):716–23.
37. Boultwood J, Pellagatti A, McKenzie AN, Wainscoat JS. Advances in the 5q- syndrome. Blood. 2010;116(26):5803–11.

mTOR Inhibitors, with Special Focus on Temsirolimus and Similar Agents

Teresa Calimeri and Andrés J. M. Ferreri

Abstract The mammalian target of rapamycin (mTOR) is a highly conserved serine/threonine kinase that belongs to the family of PI3K-related protein kinases (PIKKs). Dysregulation of mTOR signaling is associated with the development of cancers, including myeloid and lymphoid malignancies. Here, we will provide a brief overview of mTOR inhibitors and discuss the results obtained using these compounds in hematologic malignancies and especially in lymphomas. Moreover, mechanisms of drug resistance will be highlighted.

Keywords Everolimus (RAD001) · Lymphoid Malignancies · mTOR inhibitors · Rapamycin · Ridaforolimus (MK-8669) · Temsirolimus (CCI-779)

Introduction: Rapamycin and Rapalogs History

mTOR inhibitors comprise different compounds which have been developed starting from rapamycin, a macrolide antibiotic produced by the bacterium *Streptomyces hygroscopicus*. Rapamycin was isolated in a soil sample on Easter Island, also known as Rapa Nui, from where its name is derived [1] and firstly used as an antifungal agent [2]. However, shortly after, it was also shown to have strong immunosuppressive and antiproliferative properties due to its ability to inhibit mTOR [3–5]. Thus, FDA-approved Rapamycin use in transplantation to prevent allograft rejection and in coronary-artery stents to prevent restenosis in 1999 and 2003, respectively [6]. On the other hand, its application in cancer therapy started in the late 1990s, when several analogs of the drug, called rapalogs and including temsirolimus (CCI-779), everolimus (RAD001), and ridaforolimus (MK-8669), were developed with the aim to improve its pharmacokinetics and stability (Fig. 1) [7]. Temsirolimus was the first

T. Calimeri (✉) · A. J. M. Ferreri
Unit of Lymphoid Malignancies, Department of Onco-Hematology, IRCCS San Raffaele Scientific Institute, Milan, Italy
e-mail: calimeri.teresa@hsr.it

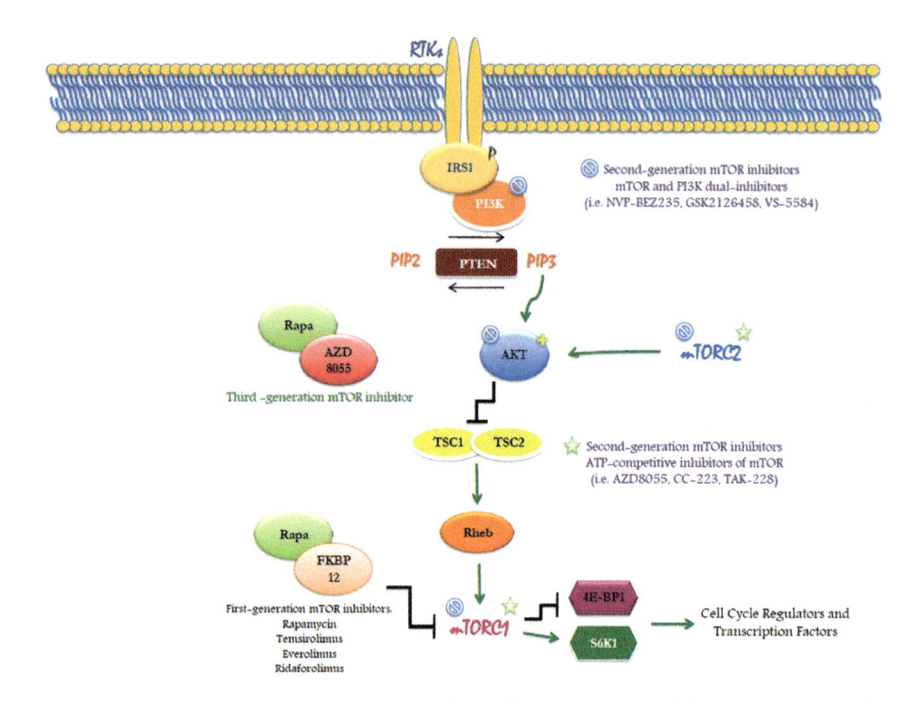

Fig. 1 Schematic representation of mTOR signaling pathways and mTOR inhibitors mechanisms of action. mTOR works through two distinct multiprotein complexes, mTOR complex 1 (mTORC1) and mTOR complex 2 (mTORC2). mTORC1 has 4E–BP1 and S6 K1 as its two major substrates by which promote the translation of key cell cycle regulators and transcription factors. mTORC2 is a key regulator of Akt full activation via phosphorylation of Ser473. Rapamycin interaction with the intracellular receptor FKBP12 as well as new generation mTOR inhibitor has been shown. The third-generation mTOR inhibitor is a molecule in which rapamycin is cross-linked with a kinase inhibitor of mTOR. Abbreviations: mTOR mammalian target of rapamycin, RTKs Receptor tyrosine kinases, PI3K phosphoinositide 3-kinase, TSC tuberous sclerosis, Rapa Rapamycin

mTOR inhibitor to gain FDA authorization for any malignancy, having been approved for the treatment of advanced renal cell carcinoma [8]. Moreover, temsirolimus is the only mTOR inhibitor approved for the treatment of lymphomas and in particular it is registered for the treatment of relapsed and/or refractory mantle cell lymphoma (MCL) in the European Union and several other countries. To date, all these agents, and the so called second generation mTOR inhibitors, are being investigated alone or in combination in solid as well as in hematologic malignancies.

The mTOR Pathway and mTOR Inhibitors

mTOR is a downstream effector of the PI3K/AKT pathway (Fig. 1). mTOR works through two distinct multiprotein complexes, mTOR complex 1 (mTORC1) and mTOR complex 2 (mTORC2) [9] which are evolutionarily conserved from yeast to mammals [10, 11]. These two complexes consist of unique mTOR-interacting proteins that determine their substrate specificity and localize them to different subcellular compartments, thus affecting their activation and function [12].

mTORC1 recruits substrates through the regulatory-associated protein of mTOR (RAPTOR) that are then further aligned to the catalytic cleft of mTOR. Rapamycin inhibits mTOR complex 1 (mTORC1) through the interaction with the intracellular receptor FKBP12 forming an inhibitory complex, which binds a region in the C terminus of TOR proteins [13, 14]. However, the exact mechanism of how this interaction with the FRB domain leads to inhibition of mTOR signaling remains to be defined. It has been proposed that rapamycin does not inhibit initial substrate recruitment but blocks correct alignment of some substrates to the catalytic cleft [15]. This could explain why rapamycin is more effective in blocking the phosphorylation and activation of ribosomal protein S6 kinase 1 (S6 K1) than that of eIF4E–binding protein 1 (4E–BP1). On the other hand, mTORC2 was identified as a rapamycin-insensitive entity, as acute exposure to rapamycin did not affect mTORC2 activity or Akt phosphorylation. However, subsequent studies have shown that, at least in some cell lines, prolonged exposure with rapamycin seems to prevent also mTORC2 assembly by progressive sequestration of the intracellular pool of mTOR and subsequently led to inhibition of AKT-signaling [16].

Temsirolimus (CCI-779), everolimus (RAD001), and ridaforolimus (MK-8669) are rapamycin analogs, called rapalogs, developed to overcome its limited pharmacological properties, such as poor water solubility and chemical stability [7] and to obtain drugs with improved pharmacokinetic (PK) properties and reduced immunosuppressive effects. However, they preserve the interactions with FKBP12 and mTOR maintaining a similar mechanism of action based on inhibition of mTORC1 and induction of cell cycle arrest in the G1 phase [17]. Unluckily, in clinical trials conducted in cancer patients they showed only limited benefits. Possible explanations could be not only due to the incomplete block of mTORC1 kinase towards its substrate 4E–BP1 and the rapalog's inability to effectively inhibit mTORC2, but also related to the existence of feedback loops as well as the activation of mechanisms outside the mTOR pathway [18].

Besides rapalogs, second generation mTOR inhibitors have been developed with the aim to have a more potent anticancer activity (Table 1). One class is represented by the so-called selective mTORC1/2 inhibitors which are small molecules working like ATP-competitive inhibitors of mTOR. In particular, they block the phosphorylation of all known downstream targets of both mTORC complexes without inhibiting other kinases. It seems that the greater anti-proliferative and pro-apoptotic effects of these molecules compared to rapamycin and observed in preclinical studies are linked to the complete block of 4E–BP1 phosphorylation and to the decreased protein expression of cyclin D1 and D3 as well as to a significant induction of p27 [19, 20]. Another class of small molecules able to inhibit mTOR is the mTOR and PI3K dual-inhibitors. With respect to the other compounds they do have the advantage to target all the three key enzymes,

Table 1 Second generation mTOR inhibitors

Compound	Company	Generic name	Phase	Disease	Mechanism of action
AZD8055	AstraZeneca		I–II	AST, GBM, HCC, Lymphomas	Selective mTORC1/2 inhibitors
CC-223	Celgene		I–II	AST, NSCLC, DLBCL	Selective mTORC1/2 inhibitors
MLN0128, INK128, TAK-228	Intellikine	Sapanisertib	I–II	AST, Lymphoma, ALL, MM, WM	Selective mTORC1/2 inhibitors
OSI-027	OSI pharmaceuticals		I	AST, Lymphomas	Dual PI3K/mTOR inhibitors
NVP-BEZ235	Novartis	Dactolisib	I–II	Breast, Renal, Prostate, GBM, Sarcoma, Pancreatic, Leukemia	Dual PI3K/mTOR inhibitors
Pf-05212384 (PKI-587)	Pfizer	Gedatolisib	I–II	Breast, Colorectal, AST, AML/MDS	Dual PI3K/mTOR inhibitors
XL147 (SAR245408)	Exelixis/Sanofi-Aventis	Pilaralisib	I–II	Breast, lung, endometrial, GBM, lymphomas	Dual PI3K/mTOR inhibitors
XL765 (SAR245409)	Exelixis/Sanofi-Aventis	Voxtalisib	I–II	Breast, lung, GBM	Dual PI3K/mTOR inhibitors
GDC-0980	Genentech	Apitolisib	I–II	Breast, renal, endometrial, colorectal, prostate, lymphomas	Dual PI3K/mTOR inhibitors

AST advanced solid tumors, *GBM* glioblastoma multiforme, *HCC* hepatocellular carcinoma, *NSCLC* non-small cell lung cancer, *DLBCL* diffuse large B-cell lymphoma, *AML/MDS* acute myeloid leukemia/myelodysplastic syndrome, *ALL* acute lymphoblastic leukemia, *MM* multiple myeloma, *WM* Waldenstrom Macroglobulinemia

PI3K, Akt, and mTOR. Thus, they potentially overcome the known feedback loops occurring with rapalogs and being active in tumors with alterations downstream of PI3K but upstream of mTOR [21]. Unluckily, the results in clinical trials are not consistent with the ones obtained in preclinical studies carried out in several types of cancers using these molecules [22].

Recently, mTOR resistance mutations to both rapalogs and kinase inhibitors of mTOR have been identified. To overcome this resistance, a third generation mTOR inhibitors have been developed. This compound was called Rapalink in order to create a bivalent interaction that exploits the unique juxtaposition of two drug-binding pockets that contain rapamycin cross-linked with a kinase inhibitor of mTOR in the same molecule [23].

Pharmacokinetics of Rapalogs

Rapamycin and rapalogs have complex pharmacokinetics [24]. The use of rapamycin in cancer treatment has been largely limited by its intrinsic chemical stability. Thus, rapamycin chemical structure has been modified to increase its water solubility and bioavailability by adding a moiety at position C43. In particular an ester, an ether, or a phosphonate group creates temsirolimus, everolimus, and ridaforolimus, respectively (Fig. 2).

Rapamycin and its derivatives are substrates for the CYP3A4 pathway [25]. Temsirolimus is quickly metabolized through de-esterification in the liver to form its primary metabolite sirolimus. However, temsirolimus is not considered a prodrug for sirolimus, as both agents are pharmacologically active. Everolimus is also metabolized, mainly in the gut and liver, but even if six main metabolites have been

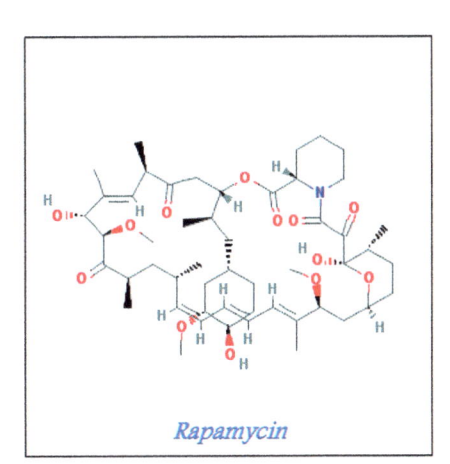

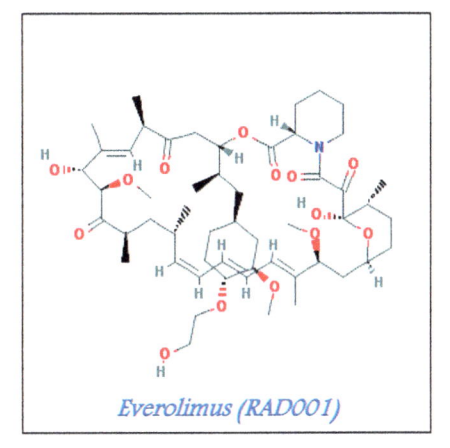

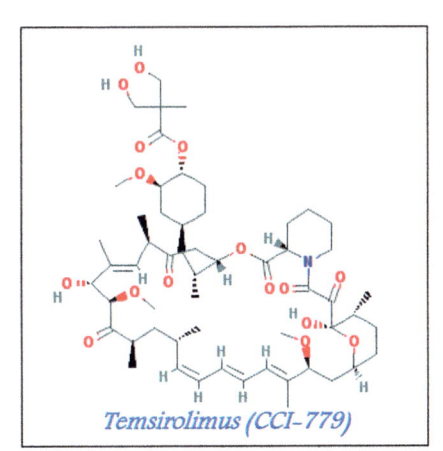

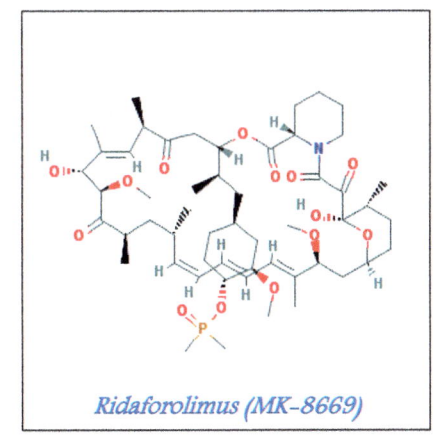

Fig. 2 Chemical structure of rapamycin and rapalogs

identified following its administration, everolimus is the main circulating component in human blood. As a result of their metabolism by isoenzymes of the CYP3A pathway, drugs that are substrates, activators, and inhibitors of these enzymes like rifampicin, anticonvulsants, and immunosuppressive compounds such as cyclosporine could potentially interact with rapalogs [26]. Moreover, due to the liver metabolism, both temsirolimus and everolimus require dose adjustments in patients with hepatic impairment while no correction is required in the presence of renal function alteration. Liver metabolism interferes also with the route of administration. Indeed, while intravenous (i.v.) rapalogs like temsirolimus and ridaforolimus display predictable pharmacokinetics with a high distribution volume and low interpatient variability, the pharmacokinetics of everolimus may be subjected to first-pass metabolism in the liver as well as influenced for absorption and bioavailability by the gastrointestinal tract (i.e. expression of ATP-binding cassette membrane transporters in the gut) [27].

Toxicity

The use of mTOR inhibitors as all the anti-cancer agents has been linked to the possibility of developing adverse events (AEs) that require specific management [28]. They can be directly mediated by the mTOR inhibitors antiproliferative effect [29] or driven by their ability to block a specific pathway [30].

Pneumonitis

Pneumonitis, or interstitial lung disease (ILD), is a potential complication of mTOR inhibitors [31]. The reported incidence varies widely as a result of a non uniform diagnostic criterium and active surveillance. Two main mechanisms for the pathophysiology of mTORi-induced ILD have been proposed. First, a directly toxic effect has been suggested since pulmonary toxicity appears to be a dose-related effect. Alternatively, an immunological origin is suggested by the high numbers of CD4+ T cells and eosinophils found in the BAL fluid of patients with ILD. In particular, three mechanisms are proposed: exposition of cryptic antigens, delayed-type hypersensitivity reaction and cytokine production. The diagnosis of mTORi-induced ILD is often difficult as clinical, radiological and pathological features are nonspecific and often are not distinguishable from respiratory infections. Thus, ILD should be a diagnosis of exclusion and diagnostic work up cannot be limited to x-ray or CT-scan but needs to include bronchoalveolar lavage (BAL) and pulmonary function tests (PFT). The onset typically occurs within 2–6 months after treatment initiation. The most common symptoms of ILD are nonspecific and include dyspnea, (dry) cough, fever, fatigue, hypoxia and occasionally hemoptysis. PFTs should be performed prior to starting mTOR inhibitor therapy to confirm a normal baseline organ function. mTOR inhibitors should be avoided in patients with significant pulmonary fibrosis or severe chronic obstructive pulmonary disease. The optimal management of ILD is essential to balance the risk of iatrogenic morbidity with the maximum efficacy using mTORi in treating cancer patients.

Metabolic Adverse Events

Hyperglycemia and hyperlipidemia are the metabolic AEs registered in patients treated with mTOR inhibitors [32].

Mammalian target of rapamycin (mTOR) inhibitors are associated with a high incidence of hyperglycemia, ranging from 13% to 50%. In particular, Grade 3 to 4 hyperglycemic events occurred in 12% of patients treated with everolimus, and in 11% of patients treated with temsirolimus. The pathophysiology of mTOR inhibitor-induced hyperglycemia and new-onset diabetes mellitus (NODM) is complex and linked to the interaction between mTOR downstream target S6 K1 with growth factors, hormones, and nutrients.

mTOR inhibitors directly act on pancreatic β-cells with a reduction in glucose-stimulated insulin secretion. On the other hand, they also seem to improve peripheral insulin resistance. Preclinical data in muscle cells showed that long-term rapamycin treatment is able to promote β-oxidation of fatty acids while diminishing basal glucose transport and glycogen synthesis [33].

A similar mechanism has been proposed for hyperlipidemia. In primary cultures of rat hepatocytes, rapamycin has been shown to affect glucose uptake and glycogen synthesis switching the metabolic preference to fatty acids as a metabolic fuel, thus, stimulating lipolysis and producing high serum levels of fatty acids [34]. Another pathophysiologic mechanism through mTOR inhibitors that may cause hyperlipidemia is an impaired lipid clearance via inhibition of insulin-stimulated lipoprotein lipase (LPL) and a significant reduction in the fractional catabolic rate of very LDL apoB100 (a triglyceride-rich lipoprotein).

Levels of lipids and glucose (preferably fasting) should be performed before starting and regularly during treatment with mTOR inhibitors. In the case of onset of metabolic AEs management strategies are similar for all causes of diabetes and hyperlipidemia. Interventions such as diet, exercise, and specific drugs (lipid-lowering agents, oral antihyperglycemic agents or insulin) should be initiated based on lipids and glucose levels.

Hematological Toxicities

An alteration in the IL-10-dependent inflammatory auto-regulation seems to be responsible of mTOR inhibitor-related anemia. In particular, it may promote disruptions in iron homeostasis and gastrointestinal iron absorption as well as effects on erythroid progenitor cell differentiation and/or erythropoietin receptor-mediated proliferation [35]. Anemia is generally mild, dose-dependent, and reversible upon discontinuation of treatment. The onset is generally within a month of initiation and is sustained throughout treatment. If detected, other causes of anemia have to be screened (i.e. occult blood in stools and vitamin B12 and folate levels). Oral or intravenous iron supplementation and erythropoiesis-stimulating agents should be effective for managing mTOR inhibitor-associated anemia, if not treatment needs to be discontinued.

Thrombocytopenia and leucopenia/neutropenia have been reported with mTOR inhibitor therapy. These AEs frequently occur simultaneously and usually resolve spontaneously. Complete blood counts should be performed routinely. Management is similar to that used for chemotherapy related-hematological toxicities. Grade 3 or higher neutropenia or thrombocytopenia may require temporary interruption of mTOR.

mTOR Inhibitors Associated Stomatitis (mIAS)

The incidence of mIAS varies widely (2–78%). As reported across multiple mTOR inhibitor clinical trials, grade 3/4 toxicities occur in up to 9% of patients. mIAS typically presents as distinct, painful, ovoid, superficial ulcers surrounded by a characteristic erythematous margin and due to a direct toxic effects of mTOR inhibitors on oral and nasal mucous membranes [36]. It resembles recurrent aphthous ulceration not only in clinical presentation but also in response to therapy.

Prophylactic strategies, including oral hygiene and avoiding injury to the epithelium of the oral cavity, are recommended. Topical high-potency corticosteroids, nonsteroidal anti-inflammatory drugs (NSAIDs) and anesthetics can be used to promote healing and reduce pain, but severe resistant mIAS could require systemic corticosteroids. Moreover, if grade 2 or higher mIAS restricts oral intake of nutrients, in such cases, mTOR inhibitor dose reduction/discontinuation may be considered.

Mechanisms of Resistance

Mutations of mTOR

Similarly to what happen in patients treated with kinase inhibitors acquired resistance mutations have been reported in cells exposed to mTORC1 inhibitors [23]. The MCF-7 breast cancer cell line was exposed to high concentrations of either rapamycin or a second-generation mTOR inhibitor (AZD8055) for 3 months. Subsequent deep sequencing of the emerged resistant colonies revealed clones harbored mutations located in the FKBP12–rapamycin-binding domain (FRB domain) or in the kinase domain. The clinical relevance of these mutations is supported by a case report of a patient who acquired an identical mTOR mutation after relapse while under treatment with everolimus [37] as well as by their observation in untreated patients.

Mutations that conferred resistance to ATP-competitive inhibitors of mTOR did not alter binding of the drug to mTOR but generated a hyperactive state of the kinase that can affect both mTORC1 and mTORC2. On the other hand, some of the identified hyper-activating mutations of mTOR are associated with increased sensitivity to rapamycin, suggesting that cancer cells harboring such mutations have an mTOR-dependent proliferation pattern. Interestingly, in a case report of a primary refractory HL, damaging mutations of the *TSC2* gene was considered responsible to the increased mTOR pathway activation and, thus, to the impressive clinical response observed using everolimus [38].

Genetic and Functional Heterogeneity

Genetic tumor heterogeneity is a well know concept in cancer biology. Both immunohistochemical staining and genome sequencing have been demonstrated that cancer cells displaying a high mTOR activity coexist with cancer cells having low mTORC1 activity in the same tumor. This observation has also been extended to primary tumor and distant metastases [39]. Moreover, genetic tumor heterogeneity has been reported for proteins that belong to signaling pathways upstream to mTOR such as PI3K/AKT and Ras/Raf/MEK/MAPK pathways.

Along with genetic alterations, a functional heterogeneity has been described for downstream effectors of mTOR like S6 K1 and 4E–BP1. An in vitro study on human colorectal cancer demonstrated that phosphorylation of S6 K1 and 4E–BP1 rarely occurs in the same cancer cell but rather shows mutual exclusivity [40]. Thus, since rapalogs do not block mTORC1-mediated 4EBP1 phosphorylation of cancer cells with a phospho-S6^{low}/phospho-4E-BP1^{high} pattern might be intrinsically resistant to rapalogs despite the presence of mTORC1 activity.

Finally, mTORC activity could be affected by micro-environmental conditions like oxygen levels [41] and pH values [42]. In both cases a downregulation of mTORC1 activity is registered, thus, cancer cells xhibit an mTORC1-independent growth and are therefore resistant to mTORC1 inhibition. Of note, hypoxia not necessarily leads to mTORC1 inhibition. For example, tumor cells harboring low levels of Ataxia Telangiectasia Mutated (ATM) protein, display a paradoxically elevated mTORC1 activity in hypoxic tumor regions. In particular, ATM is the driver of a cascade comprising HIF1α and REDD1 which inactivates mTORC1 activity in a TSC1/TSC2 dependent mechanism [43].

Alternative Proliferation Pathways

There is a complex network of regulatory feedback loops responsible for limiting the proliferative signals transmitted by upstream effectors once mTORC1 is activated. Thus, once mTORC1 is inhibited, these negative feedback loops are stopped and alternative proliferation pathways like PI3K/AKT and RAS/RAF/MEK/MAPK are free to contrast the anticancer efficacy of rapalogs. This concept has been demonstrated in the preclinical setting, in which some data showed that blocking AKT or MAPK potentiated the anticancer efficacy of rapalogs [44].

Molecular Mechanisms of mTOR Activation in Lymphomas

Aberrant activation of the mTOR pathway is a marker of more aggressive disease and poorer prognosis in both Hodgkin (HL) and non-Hodgkin lymphomas (NHLs). As already discussed, this condition can be related to mTOR specific biology but it is often linked to alterations in key upstream pathway(s) [45–47].

For example, in a subset of MCL, mTOR directly mediates Cyclin D1 downregulation trough glycogen synthase kinase (GSK)-3β [46], while other authors described PTEN inactivating phosphorylation as the key mechanism responsible for the PI3K/Akt/mTOR pathway activation. Moreover, a similar mechanism has been described in HL too [48].

Activated B-cell DLBCL (ABC-DLBCL) cell lines activate S6 K1, a downstream target of mTOR, independently from Akt either through up-regulation of PIM2 or through activation by B cell receptor (BCR) signaling components [47]. Conversely, loss of PTEN has been described to correlate with the PI3K/Akt/mTOR pathway activation in germinal center B-cell-like DLBCL (GCB-DLBCL). Of note, mTOR mutations have been described in DLBCL samples [49]. Instead, phosphorylation of Akt is common in T cell lymphoma [50].

Summary of Clinical Trials

Based on the encouraging preclinical in vitro and in vivo data [51–53] clinical trials using rapalogs have been carried out in hematological malignancies and, in particular, in lymphoproliferative disorders.

Temsirolimus

Temsirolimus has been widely investigated in hematological malignancies alone or in combinations. In lymphoma setting, it has been firstly used as single agent in a phase II trial at 250 mg/m^2 weekly in 34 patients with relapsed MCL. The overall response rates (ORR) was 38% with 1 (3%) complete response (CR) and 12 (35%) partial response (PR). The median time-to-progression in all patients was 6.5 months and the duration of response for the 13 responders was 6.9 months. Hematological toxicities were the most common adverse events (AEs) with thrombocytopenia occurring in all patients and being the most frequent cause of dose reductions even if usually resolving in 1 week. Hyperglycemia, increased triglycerides, mucositis, and fatigue were also registered [54]. A lower dose of 25 mg/m^2 weekly has been evaluated in a subsequent clinical trial with the aim to reduce the previous registered events. The ORR was similar (41%) and severe thrombocytopenia was less common (100% vs. 39%) [55]. The encouraging results of these phase II trials (RR of around 40%) pave the way for a large randomized phase III trial [56] in relapsed/refractory MCL patients. The higher doses in the temsirolimus arm (175 mg weekly for 3 weeks followed by 75 mg weekly) were significantly better than the investigator's choice both in ORR (22.2% vs 2%) and progression free survival (PFS), but the results were poorer than those reported in the phase II trial. However, data were considered consistent enough to obtain the European license for this indication. Recently, it has been published another phase III trial in relapsed/refractory MCL patients in which the standard of care temsirolimus has been used as a control arm compared to ibrutinib [57]. The primary efficacy analysis showed a significant improvement in PFS and a safer profile for patients treated with ibrutinib (median PFS 14.6 months vs 6.2 months). Moreover, an independent review committee-assessed overall response rate (ORR) was significantly higher for ibrutinib (71.9% vs 40.4%; p < 0.0001) with a CR rate of 18.7% vs 1.4%, respectively. Median treatment duration was 14.4 months for ibrutinib and 3.0 months for temsirolimus. Safety profile was favorable for the ibrutinib arm too. Reported grade 3 or higher treatment-related adverse events were lower with 94 (68%) versus 121 (87%) patients involved. Moreover, less patients discontinued treatment due AEs in the ibrutinib arm (25.5% vs 6.5%). Single agent temsirolimus has also been investigated in relapsed/refractory (Rel/Ref) primary CNS Lymphoma (PCNSL). A relatively high RR (54%) was observed but PFS (median PFS 2.1 months) was comparable with other studies [58]. Of note, treatment-associated mortality was considerable (13.5%). The authors interpretation is that frequent administration of steroids before response assessment as well as compromised condition of enrolled patients could be potential confounding factors for response evaluation and outcome. The most common AEs ≥3 grade were hyperglycemia (29.7%), thrombocytopenia (21.6%), infection (19%), anemia (10.8%), and rash (8.1%). Interestingly, neither drug nor its main metabolites were found in the CSF except in one patient in the 75-mg cohort who had 2 ng/ml of temsirolimus.

Temsirolimus has been combined with different drugs in different settings.

Combination of temsirolimus and bortezomib has been assessed in heavily pretreated Multiple Myeloma [59] and B-Cell Non-Hodgkin Lymphoma [60] patients. In both studies, the enrolled subjects received i.v. bortezomib (1.6 mg/m2) weekly on days 1, 8, 15, and 22 along with i.v. temsirolimus (25 mg) weekly on days 1, 8, 15, 22, and 29 every 35 days. Fourteen of 43 (33%) MM patients had a PR or better. Moreover, the authors noted a difference in bortezomib-responsive versus refractory patients to previous treatment with bortezomib suggesting that the combination might not completely overcome resistance or re-sensitize MM cells that are resistant to the proteasome inhibitor. On the other hand, the ORR in the Lymphoma setting was 31% (12 of 39 patients; 3 CR and 9 PR) while the median PFS was 4.7 months. Although the patients with Diffuse Large B-Cell Lymphoma (DLBCL) had a low ORR, 2 heavily pretreated patients achieved a CR after 2 cycles of therapy and both maintained remission for 7 months after the completion of protocol therapy. The underlying genetic heterogeneity of DLBCL has been suggested by the authors as presumably responsible for the wide variation observed in responses. There were no unexpected toxicities from the combination. AEs were generally manageable and similar with those reported with temsirolimus and bortezomib alone, in both studies.

The incorporation of temsirolimus in the doublet rituximab/bendamustine has been recently reported in a phase I study of Rel/Ref FL and MCL [61] showing promising preliminary activity especially in MCL along with a safety profile. An objective response was observed in 14/15 patients (93%), including 5 CR (33%; all MCL). Ongoing studies are assessing the temsirolimus combination with Rituximab and DHAP in patients with Rel/Ref DLBCL (NCT01653067) [62] and temsirolimus plus lenalidomide in relapsed NHLs (NCT01076543).

Everolimus

Like temsirolimus, the oral drug everolimus has been used as single agent in Rel/Ref aggressive and indolent NHLs [53, 63–65] as well as HL [66]. Recently, a phase II study has been carried out using oral single-agent everolimus in relapsed/refractory indolent lymphomas, mostly chronic lymphocytic leukemia (CLL) and follicular lymphoma (FL) [67]. Eligible patients received oral everolimus 10 mg daily on a 28 day-cycle schedule. The ORR in all 55 patients was 35% (19/55) with 4% (2/55) CRu, and 31% (17/55) PR; 36% (20/55) had stable disease. The median time to response was 2.3 months (range, 1.4–14.1) and the median DR was 11.5 months (95% CI, 5.7–30.4). The ORR was higher in FL (61%) than in CLL/SLL (19%). The median PFS and OS were 7.2 months and 29.4 months, respectively. Everolimus was well-tolerated with modest hematologic toxicity. Of note, two patients died of sepsis related to the drug. Thus, the authors concluded by suggesting further studies with mTORC1 inhibitors such as everolimus as single agent, and in combination with other agents. The addition of alemtuzumab to everolimus in rel/ref CLL has been published recently too, but based on their results (33% partial responses, no complete responses) no further development of this regimen was recommended by the authors [68]. Another phase II trial evaluated the activity and safety of everolimus in Rel/Ref marginal zone lymphomas (MZLs) [69]. Thirty patients received everolimus for six cycles or until dose-limiting toxicity or progression. Twenty-four out of 30 patients were evaluable and a relevant proportion experienced side effects, resulting in dose reduction (9 patients) and/or early treatment discontinuation (10 patients). ORR was 25% (1 CR and 5 PRs). Moreover, one toxic death due to treatment-related pneumonia was recorded. Thus, due to the moderate antitumor activity and the observed toxicity, it seems that single agent everolimus has limited therapeutical space in this indolent setting. Of note, it has also been carried out a phase III trial of everolimus in monotherapy as maintenance (PILLAR-2; NCT00790036) providing 1 year of adjuvant everolimus to poor-risk (IPI] ≥3) in DLBCL patients who had achieved a CR with R-chemo. No differences have been observed in the 2-yr DFS rate (78% vs 77%) even if it seemed that everolimus had a trends toward OS and DFS in selected patient subgroups (males and IPI 4/5). However, also in this setting the responses were modest, transient and in some cases toxicity was relevant [70].

Conversely from what happened in CLL/SLL, the combination of everolimus with other drugs seems to be promising. Based on the encouraging results of the preclinical data [71] showing that combining panobinostat with the mTOR inhibitor everolimus inhibited panobinostat-induced mTOR activation and enhanced panobinostat antiproliferative effects in HL cell lines, a combination of these two drugs has been carried out in a phase I trial [72]. ORR 43% with CR 15% while the dose-limiting toxicity was thrombocytopenia (grade3/4 64%). Similarly, after a phase I trial, a phase II study of everolimus in combination with CHOP (cyclophosphamide, doxorubicin, vincristine, and prednisone) as a first-line treatment for patients with peripheral T-cell lymphoma (PTCL) has been published [73]. Five (5) mg everolimus per day from day 1 to 14 every 21 days for a total of six cycles has been administered. A difference in the CR rate among subtypes was observed and was associated with PTEN loss evaluated by immunohistochemistry. Objective response rate was very high (90%; CR (n = 17) and PR (n = 10)).

Another combination has been tested in a phase I/II trial in which everolimus has been added to rituximab with or without bortezomib in Rel/Ref Waldenström's Macroglobulinemia (WM) [74]. Forty-six patients have received six cycles of both the combinations followed by maintenance with everolimus until progression. Thirty-six (78%) of the 46 patients enrolled received full dose therapy (FDT) of the three drugs. Promising results that deserve to be assessed in future trials on a larger randomized trial has been showed with an ORR of 89% (32/36 patients) with two CR (6%) and 19 PR or better response (53%). No dose-limiting toxicities have been observed in the phase I of the trial. No unexpected toxicities was recorded. Moreover, of note, 98% of registered patients had previously received rituximab, and 57% had received bortezomib.

Ridaforolimus

Only two clinical trials need to be cited on Ridaforolimus. In the first one drug has been investigated in a phase II clinical trial as monotherapy in 55 patients with Rel/Ref hematological malignancies. Drug was used as 30-min infusion on days 1–5 of a 2 weeks cycle. Of note best response was PR and it was observed only in two subsets of hematological malignancy, 29% in agnogenic myeloid metaplasia (AMM) and 33% in MCL. The most frequent grade 3/4 AEs were similar to those observed with other mTOR inhibitors, in particular mouth sores (15%), thrombocytopenia (15%), hyponatremia (7%) and hypokalemia (6%) [75]. On the other hand, the second one is a phase I study in which ridaforolimus is evaluated in combination with vorinostat in patients with advanced solid tumors or lymphoma (NCT01169532).

Second Generation mTOR Inhibitors

AZD8055 is a first-in-class dual mTORC1/mTORC2 inhibitor. In preclinical models it was shown to prevent the mTORC2-mediated AKT activation observed with rapalogs [76]. In a phase I study of 49 patients with advanced solid tumors or lymphomas (NCT00731263) [77]. MTD was 90 mg BID. The most frequent AEs were elevated transaminases (22%) and fatigue (16%). Interestingly, metabolic AEs like hypercholesterolemia nor hypertriglyceridemia were not registered as observed with other mTORC1/mTORC2 inhibitors [78, 79]. The best response was SD in 7 patients for ⩾4 months.

The results of Part A of a phase I/II study on the dual mTORC1/mTORC2 kinase inhibitor CC-223 in 28 pretreated patients with advanced solid tumors or MM has been recently published [78]. The MTD was 45 mg/d, although 11.1% of patients at the MTD required dose reductions and 55.6% required interruptions. Hyperglycemia was the most common grade 3 AE (18%). Substantial pS6 K1 (>70%), p4E–BP1 (>40%), and pAKT (>50%) inhibition was observed at ≥30 mg CC-223, although pS6 K1 and pAKT inhibition was more complete than p4E–BP1 inhibition. Additionally, preliminary evidence of inhibition of pS6 K1, p4E–BP1, pAKT, and proliferation marker Ki-67 was observed in paired tumor biopsies in 2 patients. The authors reported one PR (3.6%) lasting 220 days in 1 patient with breast cancer and 8 patients (29%) with SD (>100 days in 5 patients), including 2 patients with tumors exhibiting molecular abnormalities associated with mTORC pathway activation. Part B focused on dose expansion into parallel cohorts of selected tumor types (MM, DLBCL, and selected solid tumors) is ongoing (NCT01177397).

TAK-228, another dual mTORC1/mTORC2 kinase inhibitor, has been tested in a phase I study including 39 patients with MM (31), NHL (4), and WM (4) [79]. Drug has been administered once daily (QD) at 2, 4, 6, or 7 mg, or QD for 3 days on and 4 days off each week (QDx3d QW) at 9 or 12 mg, in 28-day cycles. Cycle 1

DLTs occurred in 5 QD patients (stomatitis, urticaria, blood creatinine elevation, fatigue, and nausea and vomiting) and 4 QDx3d QW patients (erythematous rash, fatigue, asthenia, mucosal inflammation, and thrombocytopenia). The MTDs were determined to be 4 mg QD and 9 mg QDx3d QW. Thirty-six patients (92%) reported at least one drug-related toxicity; the most common grade ≥3 drug-related toxicities were thrombocytopenia (15%), fatigue (10%), and neutropenia (5%). Of the 33 response-evaluable patients, one MM patient had a minimal response, one WM patient achieved PR, one WM patient had a minor response, and 18 patients (14 MM, 2 NHL, and 2 WM) had SD. Authors concluded saying that further studies including combination strategies need to be carried out.

Preliminary data on BEZ235, a dual PI3-Kinase/mTOR inhibitor in adult patients with RR acute leukemia showing a single-agent anti-leukemic efficacy most pronounced in ALL, with an overall response rate of 30% and a sustained molecular remission in one patient. Since results of PK analysis and assessment of PD markers associated with PI3K signaling did not correlate with response the authors concluded that a more comprehensive genomic analysis may help to identify a subset of patients likely to benefit from treatment with dual PI3K-mTOR inhibitors (NCT01756118) [80].

CC-115, a novel inhibitor of mTOR kinase and DNA-PK, was evaluated in primary CLL cells in vitro and in seven Rel/Ref CLL patients and one SLL patient harboring ATM deletions/mutations enrolled in a larger phase I clinical trial, including 110 additional patients with solid tumors (NCT01353625) [81]. All but one patient had a decrease in lymphadenopathy, resulting in one iwCLL partial response (PR) and three PRs with lymphocytosis. Moreover, the encouraging preclinical data on the ability of CC-115 to revert CD40-mediated resistance to chemotherapy or venetoclax as well as to overcome Idelalisib resistance makes this compound attractive for further combination studies in the clinical setting.

Summary

The PI3K/AKT/mTOR signaling pathway plays a central role in cell growth proliferation and survival controlling different processes in protein synthesis and angiogenesis. Deregulation of this pathway is commonly found in several types of tumors.

Currently, two mTOR inhibitors, everolimus and temsirolimus, are approved by the European Medicines Agency (EMA) and the US Food and Drug Administration to treat cancer patients in clinical practice.

Unluckily the promising results obtained in the preclinical settings using rapalogs did not translate into the expected benefits in clinical trials because response to mTOR inhibitors is not durable and patients ultimately progress because of various mechanisms of resistance. The so-called "second generation mTOR inhibitors" are small molecules developed with the aim to overcome rapalogs weaknesses. However clinical trials results do not seems to differ a lot from those obtained with rapalogs.

Common and serious mTOR inhibitors related side effects include non-infectious pneumonitis, metabolic disorders, hematological and mucosal toxicities. They require specific management in order to balance risk and benefit related to the specific treatment.

Looking forward correlative or translational sub-studies are needed to clearly and quickly identify biomarkers of response and emerging drug resistance in order to maximize the benefit linked to mTOR inhibitors treatment. Moreover, future approaches may consider combinational strategies as a way to overcome such resistance and therefore improve efficacy of mTOR targeting agents in the clinical context.

References

1. Vézina C, Kudelski A, Sehgal SN. Rapamycin (AY-22,989), a new antifungal antibiotic. I. Taxonomy of the producing streptomycete and isolation of the active principle. J Antibiot (Tokyo). 1975;28(10):721–6.
2. Sehgal SN, Baker H, Vézina C. Rapamycin (AY-22,989), a new antifungal antibiotic. II. Fermentation, isolation and characterization. J Antibiot (Tokyo). 1975;28:727–32.
3. Eng CP, Sehgal SN, Vézina C. Activity of rapamycin (AY-22,989) against transplanted tumors. J Antibiot (Tokyo). 1984;37(10):1231–7.
4. Yatscoff RW, LeGatt DF, Kneteman NM. Therapeutic monitoring of rapamycin: a new immunosuppressive drug. Ther Drug Monit. 1993;15(6):478–82.
5. Guertin DA, Sabatini DM. Defining the role of mTOR in cancer. Cancer Cell. 2007;12(1):9–22.
6. Abizaid A. Sirolimus-eluting coronary stents: a review. Vasc Health Risk Manag. 2007;3(2):191–201.
7. Ballou LM, Lin RZ. Rapamycin and mTOR kinase inhibitors. J Chem Biol. 2008;1(1–4):27–36.
8. Baldo P, Cecco S, Giacomin E, Lazzarini R, Ros B, Marastoni S. mTOR pathway and mTOR inhibitors as agents for cancer therapy. Curr Cancer Drug Targets. 2008;8(8):647–65.
9. Laplante M, Sabatini DM. mTOR signaling in growth control and disease. Cell. 2012;149(2):274–93.
10. Helliwell SB, Wagner P, Kunz J, Deuter-Reinhard M, Henriquez R, Hall MN. TOR1 and TOR2 are structurally and functionally similar but not identical phosphatidylinositol kinase homologues in yeast. Mol Biol Cell. 1994;5(1):105–18.
11. Loewith R, Jacinto E, Wullschleger S, Lorberg A, Crespo JL, Bonenfant D, Oppliger W, Jenoe P, Hall MN. Two TOR complexes, only one of which is rapamycin sensitive, have distinct roles in cell growth control. Mol Cell. 2002;10(3):457–68.
12. Betz C, Hall MN. Where is mTOR and what is it doing there? J Cell Biol. 2013;203(4):563–74.
13. Chen J, Zheng XF, Brown EJ, Schreiber SL. Identification of an 11-kDa FKBP12-rapamycin-binding domain within the 289-kDa FKBP12-rapamycin-associated protein and characterization of a critical serine residue. Proc Natl Acad Sci U S A. 1995;92(11):4947–51.
14. Choi J, Chen J, Schreiber SL, Clardy J. Structure of the FKBP12-rapamycin complex interacting with the binding domain of human FRAP. Science. 1996;273(5272):239–42.
15. Shimobayashi M, Hall MN. Making new contacts: the mTOR network in metabolism and signalling crosstalk. Nat Rev Mol Cell Biol. 2014;15(3):155–62.
16. Sarbassov DD, Ali SM, Sengupta S, Sheen JH, Hsu PP, Bagley AF, Markhard AL, Sabatini DM. Prolonged rapamycin treatment inhibits mTORC2 assembly and Akt/PKB. Mol Cell. 2006;22(2):159–68.
17. Fingar DC, Blenis J. Target of rapamycin (TOR): an integrator of nutrient and growth factor signals and coordinator of cell growth and cell cycle progression. Oncogene. 2004;23(18):3151–71.

18. Calimeri T, Ferreri AJM. M-TOR inhibitors and their potential role in haematological malignancies. Br J Haematol. 2017;177(5):684–702.
19. Mi W, Ye Q, Liu S, She QBAKT. Inhibition overcomes rapamycin resistance by enhancing the repressive function of PRAS40 on mTORC1/4E-BP1 axis. Oncotarget. 2015;6(16):13962–77.
20. Thoreen CC, Kang SA, Chang JW, Liu Q, Zhang J, Gao Y, Reichling LJ, Sim T, Sabatini DM, Gray NS. An ATP-competitive mammalian target of rapamycin inhibitor reveals rapamycin-resistant functions of mTORC1. J Biol Chem. 2009;284(12):8023–32.
21. Dienstmann R, Rodon J, Serra V, Tabernero J. Picking the point of inhibition: a comparative review of PI3K/AKT/mTOR pathway inhibitors. Mol Cancer Ther. 2014;13(5):1021–31.
22. Rodon J, Dienstmann R, Serra V, Tabernero J. Development of PI3K inhibitors: lessons learned from early clinical trials. Nat Rev Clin Oncol. 2013;10(3):143–53.
23. Rodrik-Outmezguine VS, Okaniwa M, Yao Z, Novotny CJ, McWhirter C, Banaji A, Won H, Wong W, Berger M, de Stanchina E, Barratt DG, Cosulich S, Klinowska T, Rosen N, Shokat KM. Overcoming mTOR resistance mutations with a new-generation mTOR inhibitor. Nature. 2016;534(7606):272–6.
24. Danesi R, Boni JP, Ravaud A. Oral and intravenously administered mTOR inhibitors for metastatic renal cell carcinoma: pharmacokinetic considerations and clinical implications. Cancer Treat Rev. 2013;39(7):784–92.
25. Klümpen HJ, Beijnen JH, Gurney H, Schellens JH. Inhibitors of mTOR. Oncologist. 2010;15(12):1262–9.
26. Boni J, Leister C, Burns J, Cincotta M, Hug B, Moore L. Pharmacokinetic profile of temsirolimus with concomitant administration of cytochrome p450-inducing medications. J Clin Pharmacol. 2007;47(11):1430–9.
27. Kirchner GI, Meier-Wiedenbach I, Manns MP. Clinical pharmacokinetics of everolimus. Clin Pharmacokinet. 2004;43(2):83–95.
28. Kaplan B, Qazi Y, Wellen JR. Strategies for the management of adverse events associated with mTOR inhibitors. Transplant Rev (Orlando). 2014;28(3):126–33.
29. Mahé E, Morelon E, Lechaton S, Sang KH, Mansouri R, Ducasse MF, Mamzer-Bruneel MF, de Prost Y, Kreis H, Bodemer C. Cutaneous adverse events in renal transplant recipients receiving sirolimus-based therapy. Transplantation. 2005;79(4):476–82.
30. Houde VP, Brûlé S, Festuccia WT, Blanchard PG, Bellmann K, Deshaies Y, Marette A. Chronic rapamycin treatment causes glucose intolerance and hyperlipidemia by upregulating hepatic gluconeogenesis and impairing lipid deposition in adipose tissue. Diabetes. 2010;59(6):1338–48.
31. Willemsen AE, Grutters JC, Gerritsen WR, van Erp NP, van Herpen CM, Tol J. mTOR inhibitor-induced interstitial lung disease in cancer patients: comprehensive review and a practical management algorithm. Int J Cancer. 2016;138(10):2312–21.
32. Busaidy NL, Farooki A, Dowlati A, Perentesis JP, Dancey JE, Doyle LA, Brell JM, Siu LL. Management of metabolic effects associated with anticancer agents targeting the PI3K-Akt-mTOR pathway. J Clin Oncol. 2012;30(23):2919–28.
33. Di Paolo S, Teutonico A, Leogrande D, Capobianco C, Schena PF. Chronic inhibition of mammalian target of rapamycin signaling downregulates insulin receptor substrates 1 and 2 and AKT activation: a crossroad between cancer and diabetes? J Am Soc Nephrol. 2006;17(8):2236–44.
34. Kraemer FB, Takeda D, Natu V, Sztalryd C. Insulin regulates lipoprotein lipase activity in rat adipose cells via wortmannin- and rapamycin-sensitive pathways. Metabolism. 1998;47(5):555–9.
35. Sofroniadou S, Kassimatis T, Goldsmith D. Anaemia, microcytosis and sirolimus--is iron the missing link? Nephrol Dial Transplant. 2010;25(5):1667–75.
36. Peterson DE, O'Shaughnessy JA, Rugo HS, Elad S, Schubert MM, Viet CT, Campbell-Baird C, Hronek J, Seery V, Divers J, Glaspy J, Schmidt BL, Meiller TF. Oral mucosal injury caused by mammalian target of rapamycin inhibitors: emerging perspectives on pathobiology and impact on clinical practice. Cancer Med. 2016;5(8):1897–907.

37. Wagle N, Grabiner BC, Van Allen EM, Amin-Mansour A, Taylor-Weiner A, Rosenberg M, Gray N, Barletta JA, Guo Y, Swanson SJ, Ruan DT, Hanna GJ, Haddad RI, Getz G, Kwiatkowski DJ, Carter SL, Sabatini DM, Jänne PA, Garraway LA, Lorch JH. Response and acquired resistance to everolimus in anaplastic thyroid cancer. N Engl J Med. 2014;371(15):1426–33.
38. Perini GF, Campregher PV, Ross JS, Ali S, Hamerschlak N, Santos FP. Clinical response to everolimus in a patient with Hodgkin's lymphoma harboring a TSC2 mutation. Blood Cancer J. 2016;6:e420.
39. Gerlinger M, Rowan AJ, Horswell S, Math M, Larkin J, Endesfelder D, GronroosE MP, Matthews N, Stewart A, Tarpey P, Varela I, Phillimore B, Begum S, McDonald NQ, Butler A, Jones D, Raine K, Latimer C, Santos CR, Nohadani M, Eklund AC, Spencer-Dene B, Clark G, Pickering L, Stamp G, Gore M, Szallasi Z, Downward J, Futreal PA, Swanton C. Intratumor heterogeneity and branched evolution revealed by multiregion sequencing. N Engl J Med. 2012;366(10):883–92.
40. Gerdes MJ, Sevinsky CJ, Sood A, Adak S, Bello MO, Bordwell A, Can A, Corwin A, Dinn S, Filkins RJ, Hollman D, Kamath V, Kaanumalle S, Kenny K, Larsen M, Lazare M, Li Q, Lowes C, McCulloch CC, McDonough E, Montalto MC, Pang Z, Rittscher J, Santamaria-Pang A, Sarachan BD, Seel ML, Seppo A, Shaikh K, Sui Y, Zhang J, Ginty F. Highly multiplexed single-cell analysis of formalin-fixed, paraffin-embedded cancer tissue. Proc Natl Acad Sci U S A. 2013;110(29):11982–7.
41. Wouters BG, Koritzinsky M. Hypoxia signalling through mTOR and the unfolded protein response in cancer. Nat Rev Cancer. 2008;8(11):851–64.
42. Faes S, Duval AP, Planche A, Uldry E, Santoro T, Pythoud C, Dormond O. Acidic tumor microenvironment abrogates the efficacy of mTORC1 inhibitors. Mol Cancer. 2016;15(1):78.
43. Cam H, Easton JB, High A, Houghton PJ. mTORC1 signaling under hypoxic conditions is controlled by ATM-dependent phosphorylation of HIF-1α. Mol Cell. 2010;40(4):509–20.
44. Carracedo A, Ma L, Teruya-Feldstein J, Rojo F, Salmena L, Alimonti A, Pandolfi PP. Inhibition of mTORC1 leads to MAPK pathway activation through a PI3K-dependent feedback loop in human cancer. J Clin Invest. 2008;118(9):3065–74.
45. Abubaker J, Bavi PP, Al-Harbi S, Siraj AK, Al-Dayel F, Uddin S, Al-Kuraya K. PIK3CA mutations are mutually exclusive with PTEN loss in diffuse large B-cell lymphoma. Leukemia. 2007;21(11):2368–70.
46. Dal Col J, Zancai P, Terrin L, Guidoboni M, Ponzoni M, Pavan A, Spina M, Bergamin S, Rizzo S, Tirelli U, De Rossi A, Doglioni C, Dolcetti R. Distinct functional significance of Akt and mTOR constitutive activation in mantle cell lymphoma. Blood. 2008;111(10):5142–51.
47. Ezell SA, Wang S, Bihani T, Lai Z, Grosskurth SE, Tepsuporn S, Davies BR, Huszar D, Byth KF. Differential regulation of mTOR signaling determines sensitivity to AKT inhibition in diffuse large B cell lymphoma. Oncotarget. 2016;7(8):9163–74.
48. Dutton A, Reynolds GM, Dawson CW, Young LS, Murray PG. Constitutive activation of phosphatidyl-inositide 3 kinase contributes to the survival of Hodgkin's lymphoma cells through a mechanism involving Akt kinase and mTOR. J Pathol. 2005;205(4):498–506.
49. Zhang J, Grubor V, Love CL, Banerjee A, Richards KL, Mieczkowski PA, Dunphy C, Choi W, Au WY, Srivastava G, Lugar PL, Rizzieri DA, Lagoo AS, Bernal-Mizrachi L, Mann KP, Flowers C, Naresh K, Evens A, Gordon LI, Czader M, Gill JI, Hsi ED, Liu Q, Fan A, Walsh K, Jima D, Smith LL, Johnson AJ, Byrd JC, Luftig MA, Ni T, Zhu J, Chadburn A, Levy S, Dunson D, Dave SS. Genetic heterogeneity of diffuse large B-cell lymphoma. Proc Natl Acad Sci U S A. 2013;110(4):1398–403.
50. Cai Q, Deng H, Xie D, Lin T, Lin T. Phosphorylated AKT protein is overexpressed in human peripheral T-cell lymphomas and predicts decreased patient survival. Clin Lymphoma Myeloma Leuk. 2012;12(2):106–12.
51. Wanner K, Hipp S, Oelsner M, Ringshausen I, Bogner C, Peschel C, Decker T. Mammalian target of rapamycin inhibition induces cell cycle arrest in diffuse large B cell lymphoma (DLBCL) cells and sensitises DLBCL cells to rituximab. Br J Haematol. 2006;134(5):475–84.

52. Márk Á, Hajdu M, Váradi Z, Sticz TB, Nagy N, Csomor J, Berczi L, Varga V, Csóka M, Kopper L, Sebestyén A. Characteristic mTOR activity in Hodgkin-lymphomas offers a potential therapeutic target in high risk disease–a combined tissue microarray, in vitro and in vivo study. BMC Cancer. 2013;13:250.
53. Witzig TE, Reeder C, Han JJ, LaPlant B, Stenson M, Tun HW, Macon W, Ansell SM, Habermann TM, Inwards DJ, Micallef IN, Johnston PB, Porrata LF, Colgan JP, Markovic S, Nowakowski GS, M G. The mTORC1 inhibitor everolimus has antitumor activity in vitro and produces tumor responses in patients with relapsed T-cell lymphoma. Blood. 2015;126(3):328–35.
54. Witzig TE, Geyer SM, Ghobrial I, Inwards DJ, Fonseca R, Kurtin P, Ansell SM, Luyun R, Flynn PJ, Morton RF, Dakhil SR, Gross H, Kaufmann SH. Phase II trial of single-agent temsirolimus (CCI-779) for relapsed mantle cell lymphoma. J Clin Oncol. 2005;23(23):5347–56.
55. Ansell SM, Inwards DJ, Rowland KM Jr, Flynn PJ, Morton RF, Moore DF Jr, Kaufmann SH, Ghobrial I, Kurtin PJ, Maurer M, Allmer C, Witzig TE. Low-dose, single-agent temsirolimus for relapsed mantle cell lymphoma: a phase 2 trial in the North Central Cancer Treatment Group. Cancer. 2008;113(3):508–14.
56. Hess G, Herbrecht R, Romaguera J, Verhoef G, Crump M, Gisselbrecht C, Laurell A, Offner F, Strahs A, Berkenblit A, Hanushevsky O, Clancy J, Hewes B, Moore L, Coiffier B. Phase III study to evaluate temsirolimus compared with investigator's choice therapy for the treatment of relapsed or refractory mantle cell lymphoma. J Clin Oncol. 2009;27(23):3822–9.
57. Dreyling M, Jurczak W, Jerkeman M, Silva RS, Rusconi C, Trneny M, Offner F, Caballero D, Joao C, Witzens-Harig M, Hess G, Bence-Bruckler I, Cho SG, Bothos J, Goldberg JD, Enny C, Traina S, Balasubramanian S, Bandyopadhyay N, Sun S, Vermeulen J, Rizo A, Rule S. Ibrutinib versus temsirolimus in patients with relapsed or refractory mantle-cell lymphoma: an international, randomized, open-label, phase 3 study. Lancet. 2016;387(10020):770–8.
58. Korfel A, Schlegel U, Herrlinger U, Dreyling M, Schmidt C, von Baumgarten L, Pezzutto A, Grobosch T, Kebir S, Thiel E, Martus P, Kiewe P. Phase II trial of Temsirolimus for relapsed/refractory primary CNS lymphoma. J Clin Oncol. 2016;34(15):1757–63.
59. Ghobrial IM, Weller E, Vij R, Munshi NC, Banwait R, Bagshaw M, Schlossman R, Leduc R, Chuma S, Kunsman J, Laubach J, Jakubowiak AJ, Maiso P, Roccaro A, Armand P, Dollard A, Warren D, Harris B, Poon T, Sam A, Rodig S, Anderson KC, Richardson PG. Weekly bortezomib in combination with temsirolimus in relapsed or relapsed and refractory multiple myeloma: a multicentre, phase 1/2, open-label, dose-escalation study. Lancet Oncol. 2011;12(3):263–72.
60. Fenske TS, Shah NM, Kim KM, Saha S, Zhang C, Baim AE, Farnen JP, Onitilo AA, Blank JH, Ahuja H, Wassenaar T, Qamar R, Mansky P, Traynor AM, Mattison RJ, Kahl BS. A phase 2 study of weekly temsirolimus and bortezomib for relapsed or refractory B-cell non-Hodgkin lymphoma: a Wisconsin oncology network study. Cancer. 2015;121(19):3465–71.
61. Hess G, Keller U, Scholz CW, Witzens-Harig M, Atta J, Buske C, Kirschey S, Ruckes C, Medler C, van Oordt C, Klapper W, Theobald M, Dreyling M. Safety and efficacy of Temsirolimus in combination with Bendamustine and Rituximab in relapsed mantle cell and follicular lymphoma. Leukemia. 2015;29(8):1695–701.
62. Witzens-Harig M, Keller U, Viardot A, Buske C, Cromb A, Hoenig E, Meissner J, Ho AD, Marks R, Dreyling MH, Safety HG. Clinical activity of Temsirolimus in combination with rituximab and DHAP in patients with relapsed or refractory diffuse large B-cell lymphoma – results of the part I cohort of the STORM trial. Blood. 2015;120:2727.
63. Smith SM, van Besien K, Karrison T, Dancey J, McLaughlin P, Younes A, Smith S, Stiff P, Lester E, Modi S, Doyle LA, Vokes EE, Pro B. Temsirolimus has activity in non-mantle cell non-Hodgkin's lymphoma subtypes: the University of Chicago phase II consortium. J Clin Oncol. 2010;28(31):4740–6.
64. Zent CS, LaPlant BR, Johnston PB, Call TG, Habermann TM, Micallef IN, Witzig TE. The treatment of recurrent/refractory chronic lymphocytic leukemia/small lymphocytic lymphoma (CLL) with everolimus results in clinical responses and mobilization of CLL cells into the circulation. Cancer. 2010;116(9):2201–7.

65. Witzig TE, Reeder CB, LaPlant BR, Gupta M, Johnston PB, Micallef IN, Porrata LF, Ansell SM, Colgan JP, Jacobsen ED, Ghobrial IM, Habermann TM. A phase II trial of the oral mTOR inhibitor everolimus in relapsed aggressive lymphoma. Leukemia. 2011;25(2):341–7.
66. Johnston PB, Inwards DJ, Colgan JP, Laplant BR, Kabat BF, Habermann TM, Micallef IN, Porrata LF, Ansell SM, Reeder CB, Roy V, Witzig TE. A phase II trial of the oral mTOR inhibitor everolimus in relapsed Hodgkin lymphoma. Am J Hematol. 2010;85(5):320–4.
67. Bennani NN, LaPlant BR, Ansell SM, Habermann TM, Inwards DJ, Micallef IN, Johnston PB, Porrata LF, Colgan JP, Markovic SN, Nowakowski GS, Macon WR, Reeder CB, Mikhael JR, Northfelt DW, Ghobrial IM, Witzig TE. Efficacy of the oral mTORC1 inhibitor everolimus in relapsed or refractory indolent lymphoma. Am J Hematol. 2017;92(5):448–53.
68. Zent CS, Bowen DA, Conte MJ, LaPlant BR, Call TG. Treatment of relapsed/refractory chronic lymphocytic leukemia/small lymphocytic lymphoma with everolimus (RAD001) and alemtuzumab: a phase I/II study. Leuk Lymphoma. 2016;57(7):1585–91.
69. Conconi A, Raderer M, Franceschetti S, Devizzi L, Ferreri AJ, Magagnoli M, Arcaini L, Zinzani PL, Martinelli G, Vitolo U, Kiesewetter B, Porro E, Stathis A, Gaidano G, Cavalli F, Zucca E. Clinical activity of everolimus in relapsed/refractory marginal zone B-cell lymphomas: results of a phase II study of the International Extranodal Lymphoma Study Group. Br J Haematol. 2014;166(1):69–76.
70. Witzig TE, Tobinai K, Rigacci L, Lin T, Ikeda T, Vanazzi A, Hino M, Shi Y, Mayer J, Costa LJ, Bermudez CD, Zhu J, Belada D, Bouabdallah K, Kattan JG, Wu C, Fan J, Louveau A-L, Voi M, Cavall F. PILLAR-2: a randomized, double-blind, placebo-controlled, phase III study of adjuvant everolimus (EVE) in patients (pts) with poor-risk diffuse large B-cell lymphoma (DLBCL). J Clin Oncol. 2016;34:7506.
71. Lemoine M, Derenzini E, Buglio D, Medeiros LJ, Davis RE, Zhang J, Ji Y, Younes A. The pan-deacetylase inhibitor panobinostat induces cell death and synergizes with everolimus in Hodgkin lymphoma cell lines. Blood. 2012;119(17):4017–25.
72. Oki Y, Buglio D, Fanale M, Fayad L, Copeland A, Romaguera J, Kwak LW, Pro B, de Castro Faria S, Neelapu S, Fowler N, Hagemeister F, Zhang J, Zhou S, Feng L, Younes A. Phase I study of panobinostat plus everolimus in patients with relapsed or refractory lymphoma. Clin Cancer Res. 2013;19(24):6882–90.
73. Kim SJ, Shin DY, Kim JS, Yoon DH, Lee WS, Lee H, Do YR, Kang HJ, Eom HS, Ko YH, Lee SH, Yoo HY, Hong M, Suh C, Kim WS. A phase II study of everolimus (RAD001), an mTOR inhibitor plus CHOP for newly diagnosed peripheral T-cell lymphomas. Ann Oncol. 2016;27(4):712–8.
74. Ghobrial IM, Redd R, Armand P, Banwait R, Boswell E, Chuma S, Huynh D, Sacco A, Roccaro AM, Perilla-Glen A, Noonan K, MacNabb M, Leblebjian H, Warren D, Henrick P, Castillo JJ, Richardson PG, Matous J, Weller E, Treon SP. Phase I/II trial of everolimus in combination with bortezomib and rituximab (RVR) in relapsed/refractory Waldenstrom macroglobulinemia. Leukemia. 2015;29(12):2338–46.
75. Rizzieri DA, Feldman E, Dipersio JF, Gabrail N, Stock W, Strair R, Rivera VM, Albitar M, Bedrosian CL, Giles FJ. A phase 2 clinical trial of deforolimus (AP23573, MK-8669), a novel mammalian target of rapamycin inhibitor, in patients with relapsed or refractory hematologic malignancies. Clin Cancer Res. 2008;14(9):2756–62.
76. Chresta CM, Davies BR, Hickson I, Harding T, Cosulich S, Critchlow SE, Vincent JP, Ellston R, Jones D, Sini P, James D, Howard Z, Dudley P, Hughes G, Smith L, Maguire S, Hummersone M, Malagu K, Menear K, Jenkins R, Jacobsen M, Smith GC, Guichard S, Pass M. AZD8055 is a potent, selective, and orally bioavailable ATP-competitive mammalian target of rapamycin kinase inhibitor with in vitro and in vivo antitumor activity. Cancer Res. 2010;70(1):288–98.
77. Naing A, Aghajanian C, Raymond E, Olmos D, Schwartz G, Oelmann E, Grinsted L, Burke W, Taylor R, Kaye S, Kurzrock R, Banerji U. Safety, tolerability, pharmacokinetics and pharmacodynamics of AZD8055 in advanced solid tumours and lymphoma. Br J Cancer. 2012;107(7):1093–9.

78. Bendell JC, Kelley RK, Shih KC, Grabowsky JA, Bergsland E, Jones S, Martin T, Infante JR, Mischel PS, Matsutani T, Xu S, Wong L, Liu Y, Wu X, Mortensen DS, Chopra R, Hege K, Munster PN. A phase I dose-escalation study to assess safety, tolerability, pharmacokinetics, and preliminary efficacy of the dual mTORC1/mTORC2 kinase inhibitor CC-223 in patients with advanced solid tumors or multiple myeloma. Cancer. 2015;121(19):3481–90.
79. Ghobrial IM, Siegel DS, Vij R, Berdeja JG, Richardson PG, Neuwirth R, Patel CG, Zohren F, Wolf JL. TAK-228 (formerly MLN0128), an investigational oral dual TORC1/2 inhibitor: a phase I dose escalation study in patients with relapsed or refractory multiple myeloma, non-Hodgkin lymphoma, or Waldenström's macroglobulinemia. Am J Hematol. 2016;91(4):400–5.
80. Wunderle L, Badura S, Lang F, Wolf A, Schleyer E, Serve H, Goekbuget N, Pfeifer H, Safety BG. Efficacy of BEZ235, a dual PI3-kinase/mTOR inhibitor, in adult patients with relapsed or refractory acute leukemia: results of a phase I study. Blood. 2013;122:2675.
81. Thijssen R, Ter Burg J, Garrick B, van Bochove GG, Brown JR, Fernandes SM, Rodríguez MS, Michot JM, Hallek M, Eichhorst B, Reinhardt HC, Bendell J, Derks IA, van Kampen RJ, Hege K, Kersten MJ, Trowe T, Filvaroff EH, Eldering E, Kater AP. Dual TORK/DNA-PK inhibition blocks critical signaling pathways in chronic lymphocytic leukemia. Blood. 2016;128(4):574–83.

Inhibitors of the JAK/STAT Pathway, with a Focus on Ruxolitinib and Similar Agents

Linda M. Scott

Abstract Substantive advances in our understanding of the pathogenesis of different types of lymphoma have arisen with the advent of methodologies to interrogate the genome, epigenome, and transcriptome of tumor cells. Amongst the most frequently perturbed intracellular signaling pathways identified in lymphoma is the JAK/STAT pathway, which has also been implicated in the pathogenesis of other blood cancers. Acquired mutations may affect this pathway by activating members of the JAK and STAT families directly, by inactivating those proteins whose normal function is to deactivate the JAKs, or by establishing autocrine signaling loops that drive JAK-mediated proliferation. The utilization of inhibitors of JAK/STAT activation may therefore benefit those individuals with lymphoma that are not served adequately by conventional therapies. Two JAK inhibitors, tofacitinib and ruxolitinib, are approved for use in humans currently, whilst others are under evaluation in clinical trials, and more efficacious drugs are being developed. The nature and therapeutic potential of these compounds in the treatment of patients with lymphoma are discussed.

Keywords JAK/STAT pathway · Lymphoma · Resistance · Ruxolitinib · JAK inhibitors

The JAK/STAT Intracellular Signaling Pathway

The Janus kinase (JAK) family of cytoplasmic tyrosine kinases in vertebrates consists of four closely related members: JAK1, JAK2, JAK3 and tyrosine kinase 2 (TYK2). Each JAK protein contains distinct domains: namely, the band 4.1, ezrin,

L. M. Scott (✉)
The University of Queensland Diamantina Institute, The University of Queensland, Translational Research Institute, Brisbane, QLD, Australia
e-mail: l.scott3@uq.edu.au

radixin and moesin (FERM), src-homology-2 (SH2), JAK-homology-1 (JH1) and JAK-homology-2 (JH2) domains. The FERM and SH2 domains mediate the interactions between the JAK protein and its cytokine receptor subunit, or with positive or negative regulators of JAK kinase activity, respectively. The JH1 and JH2 domains have significant homology to various tyrosine kinases; however, the latter lack several features considered important for a functional kinase and, accordingly, are referred to as the "pseudokinase" domains. This pseudokinase domain instead suppresses the basal kinase activity associated with its JH1 or "kinase" domain [1, 2]. Each JAK protein is constitutively associated with a cytokine receptor that itself lacks an intrinsic tyrosine kinase activity. Within the hematopoietic system, these include the receptors for granulocyte colony-stimulating factor, erythropoietin, thrombopoietin, thymic stromal lymphopoietin, the type-1 (α, β) and type-2 (γ) interferons (IFNs), and numerous interleukins (ILs). Each of these receptors utilizes different JAK combinations for intracellular signal transduction: the erythropoietin receptor utilizes JAK2 exclusively, whereas the IL2, IL4, IL7, IL9 and IL15 receptors activate JAK1 through their ligand-specific α chain and JAK3 via their common γ chain (Fig. 1a). Additional signaling diversity is provided by the differential use of activated STATs by receptor/JAK combinations; for example, whereas the IL2 and IL4 receptors both signal via a JAK1 and JAK3 pairing, IL2R activation induces homodimerization of STAT3 and STAT5, and IL4R activation induces homodimerization of STAT6.

In a cytokine-free environment, the JAK proteins are constitutively bound to their cytokine receptor scaffolds (Fig. 1a). Receptor engagement by its cognate ligand induces structural changes within the receptor [3], which in turn repositions the kinase and pseudokinase domains such that the two kinase domains within a JAK pairing are in close proximity, enabling auto-phosphorylation. The JAK kinase domains then phosphorylate tyrosine residues in the cytoplasmic domain of their affiliated cytokine receptors, which serve as docking sites for members of the signal-transducer-and-activator-of-transcription (STAT) transcription factor family. The recruited STAT monomers are activated by JAK-mediated phosphorylation, dimerize and translocate into the nucleus, where they enhance transcription at specific loci (Fig. 1b). In addition, JAK activation may induce the activation of other signaling pathways, such as the PI-3-kinase/AKT and MAP-kinase/ERK pathways.

Once the JAKs have been activated, they must be deactivated to prevent sustained STAT activation. Physiological inhibitors of JAK signaling often contain an SH2 domain that facilitates binding to JAK phospho-tyrosine residues, and induce either dephosphorylation or proteosomal degradation. Amongst the SH2-containing JAK inhibitors are members of the suppressors-of-cytokine-signaling (SOCS) family, the PTPN6 and PTPN11 protein tyrosine phosphatases (also known as SHP1 and SHP2, respectively), and SH2B3, a signaling adaptor protein. PTPN6, PTPN11 and SH2B3 all dephosphorylate the JAKs, albeit with different substrate preferences; PTPN6 associates with JAK1, JAK2 and TYK2, whereas PTPN11 associates with JAK1 and JAK2. SH2B3 directly interacts with JAK2, with its SH2 domain binding specifically to phospho-Y718. The SH2 domain of SOCS proteins, in contrast, binds to the catalytic centre of phosphorylated JAK

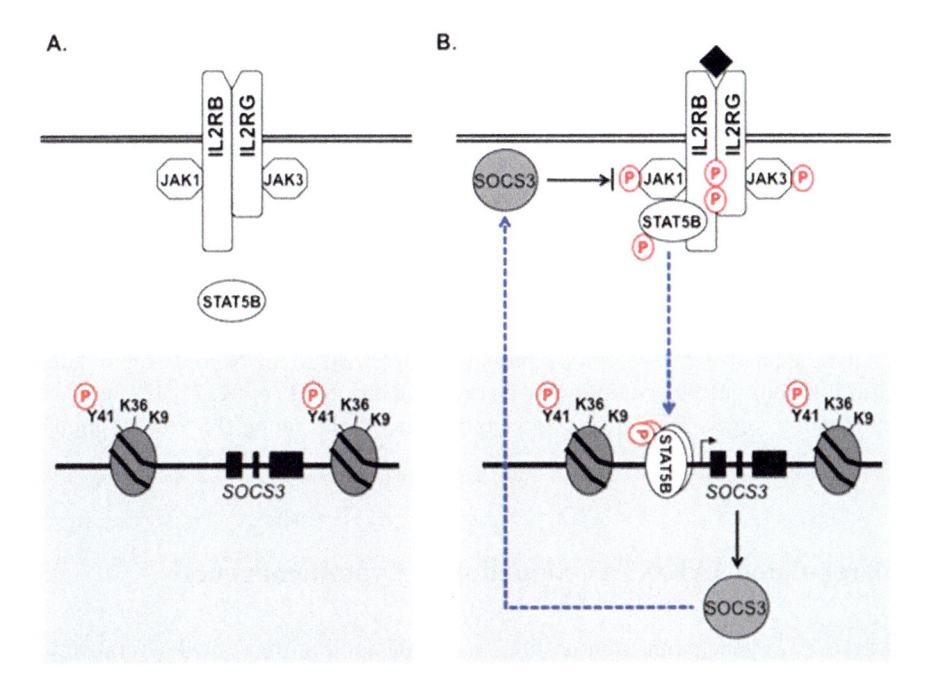

Fig. 1 *Canonical JAK/STAT signaling induced by exposure to IL2.* (**a**) In the absence of cytokine (here, IL2), JAK1 and JAK3 are tethered to their respective cytokine receptor scaffolds, IL2RB and IL2RG. (**b**) Engagement of the IL2 receptor by IL2 (depicted as a black diamond) induces structural changes within that receptor, which in turn reposition the kinase and pseudokinase domains such that the two kinase domains within a pairing are in close proximity, enabling phosphorylation in *trans*. Once auto-phosphorylated, the JAK1 and JAK3 kinase domains phosphorylates tyrosine residues in the cytoplasmic domain of the affiliated receptor chain, and these serve as docking sites for STAT transcription factors present in the cytoplasm. Recruited STAT5B monomers are activated by JAK-mediated phosphorylation, then dimerize and translocate into the nucleus, where they enhance transcription at specific loci. One STAT target gene encodes SOCS3; the SOCS proteins inhibit activated JAKs by binding to their catalytic centre. This facilitates the formation an E3 ligase complex that ubiquitinylates and marks for degradation both the JAK and the SOCS polypeptides

proteins, facilitating the recruitment of Rbx1, Cullin5, elongin-B and elongin-C to the "SOCS box" domain, thereby forming an E3 ligase complex that ubiquitinylates the JAK and SOCS polypeptides, marking them for degradation. As the SOCS proteins are downstream targets of the activated STATs, they form part of a classical negative feedback loop to limit the duration of cytokine-mediated signaling events (Fig. 1b). Phosphatases lacking an SH2 domain can also deactivate JAKs: PTPRC (known as CD45) dephosphorylates all four family members, whereas activated JAK2 or TYK2 are dephosphorylated by PTPN1, and activated JAK1 or JAK3 are dephosphorylated by PTPN2.

In addition to the canonical JAK/STAT activation, receptor engagement may cause the translocation of JAK proteins into the nucleus. Nuclear JAK2 is detectable in mammalian hematopoietic cell-lines and primary CD34⁺ progenitors [4, 5], where it phosphorylates histone H3 on Y41 (H3Y41), thereby excluding the chromo-shadow domain of the HP1α heterochromatin protein from binding to this residue. HP1α displacement leads to alterations in the chromatin structure that surrounds transcriptionally inactive genes [5, 6], including functionally important genes such as *TAL1* and *GATA2* [7]. Nuclear JAK2 can also interact with PMRT5, an arginine methyltransferase that mediates the di-methylation of arginine residues in the H2A, H3 and H4 histone proteins [8, 9]. JAK2-mediated phosphorylation of PMRT5 reduces its methyltransferase activity, altering the pattern of histone modification (9). JAK2 also phosphorylates EZH2 [10], a methyltransferase that is the catalytic subunit of the polycomb repressive complex 2 (PRC2). Non-phosphorylated EZH2 inhibits gene transcription by methylating histone H3 on K27 [11, 12]; phosphorylation targets EZH2 for degradation, thereby alleviating this transcriptional repression.

Deregulated JAK/STAT Signaling in Lymphomagenesis

Advances in gene expression profiling a decade ago has implicated several well-characterized intracellular pathways in the biology of one or more types of lymphoma; these include the NF-κB and JAK/STAT signaling pathways. For example, the molecular signatures associated with primary mediastinal B-cell lymphoma (PMBCL) and Hodgkin lymphoma (HL) include over-expression of the IL13 receptor, as well as JAK2 and STAT1 themselves [13, 14]. Use of next-generation sequencing technologies to interrogate the genomes of various types of lymphoma has more recently provided meaningful insights into their molecular etiology. Some of the mutations found to be associated with lymphoma development directly target genes that encode constituents of the JAK/STAT pathway, as summarized in Table 1, by activating positive regulators of this pathway or inactivating negative regulators. In several disorders, these mutations are not mutually exclusive and a subset of patients may have two, three or even four mutations that individually activate JAK/STAT signaling. Yet other mutations alter intracellular signaling events or gene expression patterns that directly impact upon the activation status of JAK and STAT proteins. These mutations, and their in vitro or in vivo consequences, are outlined in further details in the following sections.

Mutations that Alter JAK2 Copy Number but Not Its Coding Sequence

PMBCL and HL have a common set of pathogenetic mutations, the most well-characterized of which is a focal amplification of chromosome 9p24, which occurs in 55% of patients with PMBCL, 35% of those with HL [18–21, 44, 45], and 50%

Table 1 Gene mutations that activate JAK/STAT signaling in lymphoma cells

Gene	Lymphoma subtype	Frequency (%)	References
Activating mutations			
JAK1	EATL, type-I	50	[15]
	EATL, type-II	12	[15]
	CTCL	9	[16]
	ALK mutation –ve ALCL	15	[17]
JAK2	PMBCL	55	[18, 19]
	GZL	50	[20]
	HL	35	[21, 19]
	T-LBL	12	[22]
JAK3	EATL, type-II	33–46	[15, 23]
	NKTCL	32	[24, 25]
	ATLL	11	[26]
	CTCL	9	[16]
	- MF	10–20	[27–29]
	- Sezary syndrome	3	[30]
STAT3	EATL, type-I	25	[15]
	Cutaneous ALCL	8–20	[17, 31]
	GD-TCL	8	[32]
	NKTCL	6–11	[32, 33]
	DLBCL	3–11	[31]
	ALK- ALCL	10	[17]
	Mature TCL	4	[31]
STAT5B	EATL, type-II	36–63	[15, 23, 32]
	GD-TCL	32	[32]
	NKTCL	2–6	[32, 33]
STAT6	PMBCL	36	[34]
	Germinal center B-cell DLBCL	36	[35]
	FL	11	[36]
Inactivating mutations			
PTPN1	PMBCL	22	[37]
	cHL	20	[37]
PTPN2	PTCL	5	[38]
	HL	2	[38]
PTPN6	DLBCL	5	[39]
SH2B3	EATL, type-II	20	[15]
SOCS1	cHL	42–61	[40, 41]
	PMBCL	42	[40]
	NLPHL	50	[42]
	FL	25	[42]
	DLBCL	15–25	[42, 43]
	BL	7	[42]
	MCL	6	[42]

of those with gray zone lymphoma (GZL), an entity with features of both PMBCL and HL but which cannot readily be assigned to either classification. The common amplified region spans 3.5 Mb and twenty-one genes, ten of which are overexpressed in affected lymphoid cells [46]. Functional genetic screens showed that three genes (*RANBP6, JMJDC2, JAK2*) were required for the survival or proliferation of cells carrying this amplicon [46]; short hairpin RNA (shRNA)-mediated knockdown of JAK2 induced apoptosis, whereas proliferation was inhibited after knockdown of RANBP6 or JMJDC2. A series of elegant experiments suggests that cell viability is maintained by an autocrine signaling loop in which the expression of JAK2 is induced by IL13 and augmented by the 9p24 amplicon, resulting in phosphorylated STAT6 in the nucleus [46]. This binds to and increases the transcription of multiple genes, including *IL13*. The resultant IL13 is secreted, where it binds to IL13 receptor α (IL13RA) subunits on the lymphoma cell's surface, further enhancing intracellular JAK2 and STAT6 activation.

Given the role that JAK2 can play in epigenomic modification, Rui and colleagues evaluated the possibility that it synergizes with JMJDC2, a dioxygenase that catalyzes the demethylation of histone H3 K9 to relax regions of the epigenome that have a condensed chromatin structure [47]. JMJDC2 knockdown sensitized amplicon-positive cells to JAK2 pharmacological inhibition, confirming that these proteins co-operate to ensure the survival and expansion of lymphoma cells. Dual inhibition also increased the number of nuclear foci containing high levels of HP1α, indicating that JMJDC2 and JAK2 co-operatively suppress heterochromatin formation. Both factors modify histone H3, with JMDJC2 demethylating trimethylated K9 and K36, and JAK2 phosphorylating residue Y41. HP1α binds to these three residues and their epigenetic modification inhibits binding. Genome-wide analysis of the distribution of phosphorylated H3Y41 in amplicon-positive lymphoma cells showed that JAK2 and JMJDC2 alter transcription from numerous loci, including those encoding MYC, IL4RA, JAK2 and JMJDC2 [46]. Increased JAK2, IL4RA and JMJDC2 synthesis therefore sets up positive feedback loops that enhance IL13/JAK/STAT-mediated signaling.

Mutations that Directly Alter the JAK Family Members

Acquired activating mutations in TYK2 have not been observed in patients with lymphoma to date, although mutations targeting JAK1, JAK2 and JAK3 have been detected in a proportion of cases (Table 1).

Lymphoma-associated JAK1 mutations were first described in 4 of 46 patients with cutaneous T-cell lymphoma (CTCL), and subsequently noted in patients with ALK mutation-negative anaplastic large cell lymphoma (ALCL) or type-I or type-II enteropathy-associated T-cell lymphoma (EATL) [15–17, 48]. The JAK1 mutations associated with CTCL and EATL, type-I have not been characterized in vitro, so their effects on JAK/STAT signaling remain unclear. However, they all map to the pseudokinase domain, with most affected residues in close proximity to each other

(Y652H/N, Y654F, R659C). As the JAK1V658F mutation is activating and occurs at the analogous position to the JAK2V617F mutation [49], lymphoma-associated JAK1 substitutions may behave similarly. In contrast, all of the ALCL-associated mutations map to the JAK1 kinase domain: most affect residue G1097, although one case had a L910P mutation. G1097 substitutions were also present in 4 of 4 JAK1-mutated patients with type-II EATL [15]. When expressed in human 293-T cells, these variants induced levels of phospho-JAK1 and -STAT3 [17]. Strikingly, half of the ALCL patients with an acquired JAK1 mutation also carried an acquired STAT3 mutation (as described below); co-expression of the *JAK1* and *STAT3* mutants resulted in increased colony numbers in an in vitro colony assay, suggesting that these mutations may synergize in vivo.

Somatic JAK2 mutations occur frequently in some types of blood cancer, in particular the myeloproliferative neoplasms (MPNs) [50–54], and Down syndrome-associated and high-risk sporadic acute lymphoblastic leukemia (ALL) [55, 56]. In contrast, they occur rarely in cases of lymphoma [57–59], with a proportion of affected patients carrying chromosomal rearrangements of chromosome 9p. About 1% of patients with classical HL (cHL) carry a reciprocal t(4;9) translocation that generates a fusion protein consisting of the distal half of JAK2, and the proximal part of SEC31A, a protein implicated in vesicular transport [60]. Expression of this fusion protein produces cytokine-independent proliferation in vitro, and an aggressive T-cell lymphoblastic lymphoma (T-LBL) in vivo [60]. A TEL/JAK2 protein chimera arising from a t(4;12) translocation has also been reported in an adult patient with T-LBL [22]. Two of eight cases of pediatric T-LBL instead had acquired substitutions in the JAK2 pseudokinase domain: H574R and R683G, which is one of the JAK2 mutants present in ALL associated with Down syndrome [22]. Expression of each of the three T-LBL JAK2 mutants in vitro resulted in elevated levels of phospho-STAT5, and increased transcription of the *LMO2* gene, a known target of JAK/STAT activation.

Acquired mutations in the JAK3 pseudokinase (A572V and A573V) have been identified in 32% of patients with natural killer/T-cell lymphoma [24, 25]; these variants may also be present in cases of with mycosis fungoides, or Sezary syndrome, a leukemic variant of CTCL [16, 27–30]. Other CTCL patients have mutations elsewhere in this domain (M511I, K561I, V678 L and P745L). A sizeable proportion of patients with type-II EATL also have a JAK3A573V mutation; other patients may have a V674A, V674F or M511I mutation, or an occasional other variant (Q507P, R657W, P676R and V678 L) in the pseudokinase domain can occur [15, 23]. JAK3 mutations have not been reported in type-I EATL, but this may be due to the small number of cases assessed thus far. The A572V substitution provides an in vitro gain-of-function: BaF3 murine pro-B cells no longer require IL3 for proliferation, and contain increased levels of phospho-JAK3 and -STAT5 [25, 61]. JAK3A572V expression in primary bone marrow cells generates a fatal lymphoproliferative disorder when transplanted into mice [29].

In addition, FERM domain mutations affecting JAK3 residues L156, R172 or E183 have been detected in four of 36 patients with adult T-cell leukemia/lymphoma (ATLL) [26]. When expressed in vitro, these variants enabled cytokine-independent cell growth, with increased levels of phosphorylated JAK3 and STAT5, demonstrating that they are true gain-of-function mutations. The mechanism by which these variants activate the JAK/STAT pathway is unclear, but might be due to decreased JAK3 turnover, as they were apparently more stable in BaF3 cells than their wild-type counterpart [26].

Mutations that Target the STAT Family Members

Although mutations targeting the STAT proteins rarely occur in hematologic malignancies, studies have identified lymphoma patients with an acquired *STAT3* mutation, including those with type-I EATL, ALK mutation-negative cutaneous ALCL, natural killer/T-cell lymphoma (NKTCL), DLBCL and γδ T-cell lymphoma (GD-TCL) [15, 17, 31–33, 62, 63]. Variants detected in these lymphomas (including Y640F, N647I, D661Y, A662V and A702T) are the same as those identified in patients with large granular lymphocytic leukemia [64], and predominantly localize to the SH2 domain of STAT3, although an activating mutation in the coiled-coil domain has been described [65]. In primary lymphoma samples, the presence of a STAT3 mutation was associated with elevated levels of nuclear STAT3 [17]. Several lines of evidence together suggest these are activating mutations: their expression increased STAT3 phosphorylation, nuclear translocation and transcriptional activity in vitro [32, 64, 65], and cell-lines derived from NKTCL and GD-TCL samples that were positive for a STAT3 mutation had impaired proliferation following shRNA-mediated STAT3 knockdown [32]. Mice transplanted with bone marrow cells expressing the STAT3Y640F mutant developed blood abnormalities, although the phenotype was not lymphoproliferative but rather included transient hyperleukocytosis, anemia, and a progressive increase in platelet counts [31].

STAT5B mutations have been detected at high frequency in patients with type-I EATL and GD-TCL, and at a lower frequency in those with NKTCL [15, 23, 32, 33]. Residues N642 (within the SH2 domain) and V712 (transactivation domain) are mutation hotspots, although T628S, Q636P, Y665F, and Q706L substitutions can also occur. In primary type-I EATL samples, the presence of a STAT5 mutation was associated with elevated levels of nuclear STAT5 [23], and expression of the N642H or V712E variants in HeLa cells resulted in increases in STAT5 phosphorylation and transcriptional activity [15]. Ectopic expression of mutant STAT5B, but not wildtype STAT5B, also promoted robust proliferation of primary NK cells in vitro [32], with corresponding increased transcription of several STAT5B target genes (encoding BCL2, BCL-xL, HIF2α and IL2Rα).

Recurrent *STAT6* mutations have been identified in 36% of patients with PMBCL, and 10% of cases of FL [34, 36, 66]. Each mutation caused a substitution within the STAT6 DNA binding domain, primarily affecting N417 or D419. In vitro studies have confirmed that the mutant STAT6 proteins were constitutively activate, with their expression resulting in the transactivation of a STAT6 reporter construct in the absence of exogenous IL4 [36], although the presence of a mutation was not sufficient to cause STAT6 phosphorylation, but instead resulted in an accumulation of non-phosphorylated STAT6 in the nucleus. This, in turn, resulted in the increased transcription from loci known to be a direct STAT6 target (*CISH*, *CCL17* and *FCER2*) in primary cells sampled from patients with FL.

Mutations that Inactivate Negative Regulators of the JAK/STAT Signaling

In lymphoma patients, SOCS mutations are restricted to occurring in SOCS1, where they primarily occur as mono-allelic mutations in those with HL, PMBCL or nodular lymphocyte-predominant Hodgkin lymphoma (NLPHL) [40, 42, 67]. They are also present in a quarter of cases of follicular lymphoma (FL) or diffuse large B-cell lymphoma (DLBCL), and at lower frequencies in Burkitt lymphoma (BL), mantle cell lymphoma (MCL), or plasmacytoma [42]. About half of the SOCS1 mutations result in protein truncation by causing a frame-shift that adds a variable number of additional (nonsense) amino acids. In other instances, mutations do not perturb the reading frame, but instead result in an interstitial deletion. These can occur throughout the protein but are concentrated around the SH2 domain and SOCS box, and are predicted to inactivating by interfering with the ability of SOCS1 to bind to phosphorylated JAKs or form a functional E3 ligase complex. Accordingly, cells with a *SOCS1* mutation levels would be predicted to have higher levels of activated JAKs than those expressing wildtype SOCS1. Indeed, JAK2 turnover is impaired in the MedB-1 cell-line, which was derived from a patient with PMBCL and carries two mutated *SOCS1* alleles [68]; expression of wild-type SOCS1 within these cells reduced their rate of proliferation, with a concomitant decrease in the level of phosphorylated JAK2 and STAT5. immunohistochemical analysis of bone marrow samples from patients with cHL and a *SOCS1* mutation furthermore showed high levels of phospho-STAT5 [40]; elevated levels of phospho-STAT6 are associated with a *SOCS1* mutation in patients with NLPHL [42].

PTPN1 or PTPN2 mutations result in the sustained activation of their associated JAK proteins. Mutations that affect PTPN1 have been detected in approximately 20% of PMBCL and cHL samples [37]; these include missense, nonsense and frame-shift mutations, as well as single-residue deletions. In numerous cases, co-existing PTPN1 and SOCS1 mutations were detectable. The in vitro analysis of PTPN1 mutants revealed that they all had reduced phosphatase activity compared to wild-type PTPN1 [37], with the level of impairment dependent on the mutation present: the Q9 and R156 frame-shift mutants had less than 10% wild-type PTPN1 activity, whereas the V182D and M282 L substitutions respectively had 30% and 80% activity. As a consequence of reduced phosphatase activity, phospho-STAT6 levels induced by IL4 remain elevated. Similarly, increased levels of phosphorylated JAK1, JAK2, STAT3, STAT5 and STAT6 were observed in HL cells in which PTPN1 levels were lowered by shRNA-mediated knockdown. Immunohistochemical assessment of tissues from patients with cHL or PMBCL revealed that PTPN1 protein levels were reduced in mutation-positive cases. Bi-allelic mutations in

PTPN2 can also occasionally occur in patients with HL or T-cell non-Hodgkin lymphoma (NHL) [38]. In almost all cases, an entire *PTPN2* allele was deleted, with the other allele carrying nonsense mutations that resulted either in protein truncation, or substitutions that were predicted to disrupt an α-helix within the protein tyrosine phosphatase domain. Expression of wildtype or mutant PTPN2 in BaF3 cells showed that mutant PTPN2 is expressed at substantially lower levels than its wild-type counterpart in vitro [38]. Mutant PTPN2 expression was associated with increased levels of phospho-JAK1, and concomitant increases in the levels of phospho-STAT1 and -STAT3, but not -STAT6.

Abnormalities of PTPN11 activity have not been implicated in the pathogenesis of lymphoma. However, the *PTPN6* gene is frequently hypermethylated in cases of follicular lymphoma (FL), MCL and DLBCL [69, 70], causing constitutive STAT3 phosphorylation, and *PTPN6* point mutations have been described in 2 of 38 DLBCL patients [39]. These caused substitutions at residues 225 (N225 K) and 550 (A550V), neither of which map to the SH2 domains of PTPN6. Nevertheless, in vitro characterization showed that each mutant activates JAK/STAT signaling, with elevated levels of phosphorylated JAK3 but not JAK1, JAK2 or TYK2, and elevated levels of phosphorylated STAT3 but not STAT1, STAT5 or STAT6. Compared to cells expressing wildtype PTPN6, cells that express mutant PTPN6 had elevated levels of Mcl-1 and survivin, suggesting that acquired *PTPN6* mutations may confer a proliferative or survival advantage to lymphoid cells in vivo.

SH2B3 frame-shift mutations were recently identified in 3 of 15 patients with type-II EATL [15]. These are predicted to impair SH2B3 function, although this was not formally tested. Further studies are therefore required to determine the functional relevance of SH2B3 mutations in lymphomagenesis.

Mutations that Indirectly Activate the JAK/STAT Signaling

Lymphoma-associated mutations that target constituents of signaling networks other than the JAK/STAT pathway may nonetheless activate this pathway. An example of this phenomenon is provided by lymphoma cases in which mutations affect MYD88, an adaptor protein that activates the NF-κβ pathway following stimulation of the receptors for IL1 or IL8, or the toll-like receptors (TLR) (Fig. 2). MYD88 mutations occur in 10% of patients with gastric mucosa-associated lymphoid tissue (MALT) lymphoma, 40% of patients with the activated B-cell (ABC) DLBCL, and in 90% of patients with Waldenstrom's macroglobulinemia, a lymphoplasmacytic lymphoma [71]. In vitro studies show that, in the absence of receptor-mediated signaling, mutated MYD88 associates with the IRAK1 and IRAK4 kinases, causing IRAK1 phosphorylation by IRAK4 [72]. This then initiates a phosphorylation cascade that results in the proteosomal degradation of IκB, which enables NF-κB to translocate into the nucleus and enhances transcription from specific loci. Amongst the genes induced in this manner are those encoding IL6 and IL10 [72], the autocrine secretion of which activates JAK- and STAT3-mediated

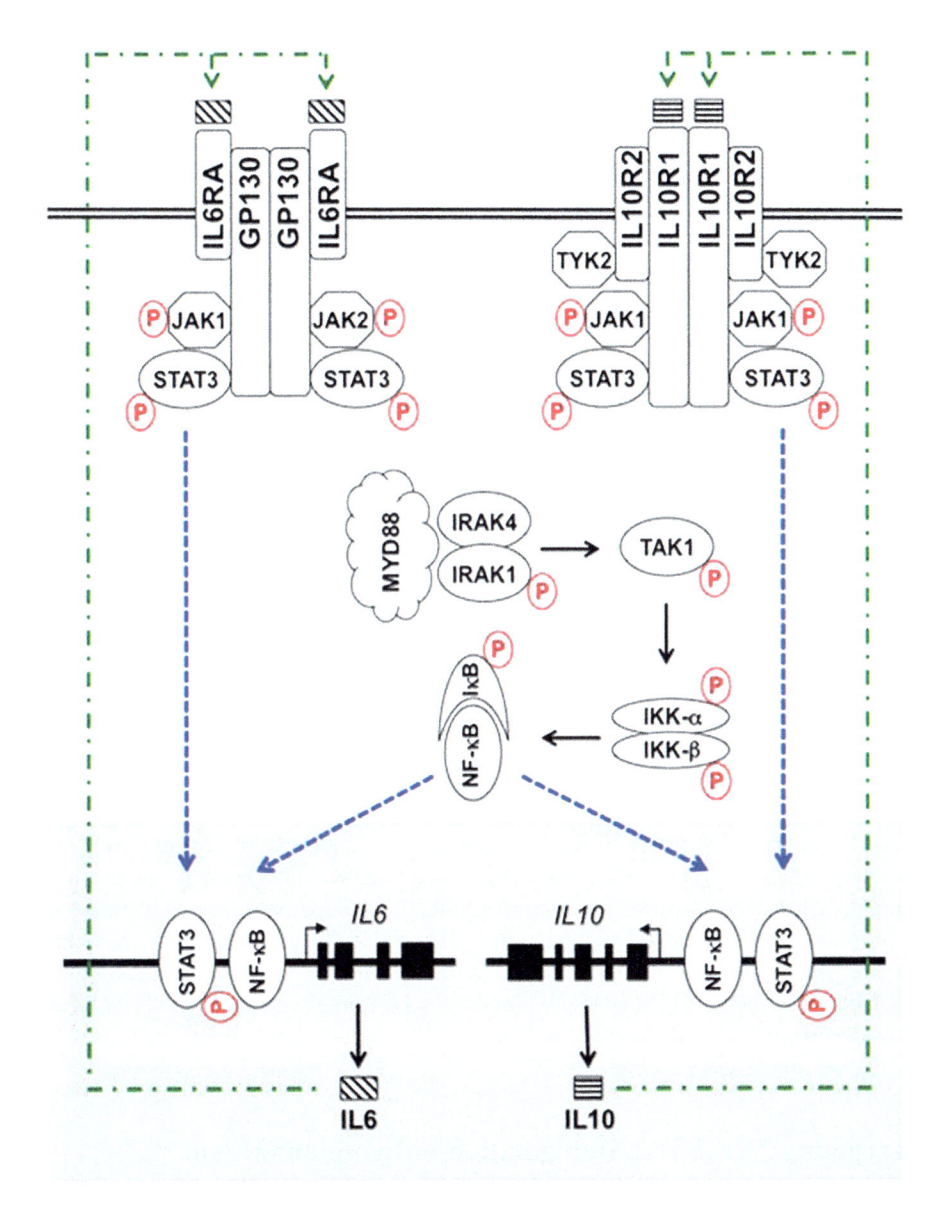

Fig. 2 *Mutation of MYD88 induces autocrine signaling mediated by IL6 and IL10.* In healthy cells, a complex consisting of MYD88, IRAK1 and IRAK4 is assembled only after MYD88 interacts with a ligand-activated TLR, or the IL1 or IL8 receptors. Mutated MYD88 (depicted by cloud shape) causes spontaneous formation of this complex. The close proximity of IRAK4 to IRAK1 in either circumstance enables phosphorylation of IRAK1, which initiates a signaling cascade involving the phosphorylation of TAK1, the IKK α and β chains, and IκB. Phosphorylation results in the ubiquitinylation and proteosomal degradation of IκB, which maintains the NF-κB transcription factor in the cytoplasm. MYD88 mutation therefore permits the nuclear translocation of NF-κB, which binds to, and enhances the transcription from, specific target genes. Amongst the loci affected are those encoding IL6 and IL10, setting up an autocrine-signaling loop that includes their cognate receptors. Signaling through either results in JAK-mediated phosphorylation and re-location of STAT3 to the nucleus, where it enhances transcription of the *IL6* and *IL10* genes, and of other functionally important genes

signaling in patients with ABC-DLBCL [73]. Therefore, the presence of a MYD88 mutation establishes a feed-forward signaling loop in which nuclear NF-κB drives the synthesis of IL6 and IL10, which are secreted into the microenvironment (Fig. 2). These then engage their cognate receptors expressed upon the lymphoma cell surface, inducing intracellular activation of JAK1, JAK2 and STAT3. Nuclear phospho-STAT3 then synergizes with NF-κβ to enhance IL6 and IL10 synthesis. This signaling loop could be disrupted, however, by exposure to OTX015, a BET bromodomain inhibitor under evaluation for the treatment of DLBCL (NCT01713582). Exposure inhibited lymphoma cell proliferation *in vitro* by inducing cell cycle arrest and apoptosis [74]. OTX015 also caused the down-regulation of genes involved in NF-κβ, TLR, and JAK/STAT signaling by displacing the bromodomain-containing protein, BRD4, from the regulatory regions of the *MYD88* gene, and reducing the levels of MYD88 protein expressed. In xenograft models of DLBCL, OTX015 treatment for 25 days results in a 60% reduction in tumor volume [74].

JAK/STAT activation also occurs as a consequence of acquired mutations in KMT2D [75], a histone lysine methyltransferase known as MLL2 or MLL4. KMT2D mutations occur in 41–89% of patients with FL, in 34% of those with nodal marginal zone lymphoma (NMZL), and in 32–39% of those with DLBCL [62, 75–77]. The nature of these mutations suggested that they were inactivating, which is supported by the observation that *KMT2D* loss in mice promotes the development of lymphoma [75]. Pathway analysis of the transcriptome associated with a KMT2D mutation revealed significant down-regulation of JAK-dependents targets, and of IL6- and IL10-induced genes, including *SOCS3* [75]. In KMT2D-wildtype OCI-LY7 lymphoma cells, shRNA-mediated KMT2D knockdown resulted in reduced transcription and translation of SOCS3, with a commensurate increase in phospho-STAT3 levels and an augmented response to IL21 exposure. The reduced transcription of *SOCS3* observed was a likely consequence of the loss of mono- and di-methylated histone H3 marks (H3K4me1 and H3K4me2) surrounding the *SOCS3* enhancer in KMT2D-deficient lymphomas.

Targeting JAK/STAT Deregulation in Lymphoma Cells

As inappropriate JAK- and STAT-mediated signaling is observed in the malignant cells of a significant number of patients diagnosed with lymphoma, the JAK/STAT pathway should be a focus for the development of novel therapies for individuals that are currently not served adequately by existing treatment regimens. These drugs may also have the potential to benefit others by limiting the toxicities associated with traditional chemotherapies. Whilst new approaches to inhibiting the activation of STAT family members are being explored in the laboratory, there are only a few investigational drugs that appear to have any clinical utility. In contrast, multiple JAK inhibitors have been evaluated in a clinical setting, with two having received US Federal Drug Administration (FDA) approval.

Table 2 Clinical trials of inhibitors of JAK/STAT signaling in lymphoma

Study drug	Target	Condition	Phase	Identifier
Ruxolitinib	JAK1/2	cHL	Ongoing	NCT02164500
		Advanced HL	II; ongoing	NCT01877005
		DLBCL, TCL	II; ongoing	NCT01431209
		Hl, PMBCL	II; ongoing	NCT01965119
		HL	II; ongoing	NCT02164500
Cerdulatinib	Pan-JAK	Aggressive NHL, FL, PTCL, CTCL	I/IIA; ongoing	NCT01994382
Ruxolitinib + bortezomib	JAK1/2	Hl NHL	I; ongoing	NCT02613598
INCB039110 + ibrutinib	JAK1/2	DLBCL	I/II; not open	NCT02760485
INCB039110 + INCB040093	JAK1/2	cHL	II; ongoing	NCT2456675
OPB-31121	STAT3	NHL	I/II; unknown	NCT00511082
AZD9150	STAT3	Lymphoma	I/II; ongoing	NCT01563302
AZD9150 + MED14736	STAT3	DLBCL	I; ongoing	NCT02549651
Pyrimethamine	STAT3	SLL	I/II; ongoing	NCT01066663

Pharmacologic Inhibitors of STAT Activation

The inhibition of STAT activity by pharmacologic drugs has proven to be challenging, with many people considering STATs and other transcription factors to be "undruggable" targets. Accordingly, there is little data published on the efficacy of STAT inhibitors in lymphoma patients, although one, OPB-31121 (Otsuka Pharmaceuticals), had a strong anti-proliferative effect on 5 of 9 DLBCL cell-lines and 3 of 3 BL cell-lines tested [78]. OPB-31121 is a small molecule STAT inhibitor that forms high-affinity interactions with the SH2 domain of STAT3. Phase I/II studies (NCT00511082; Table 2) in patients with NHL are apparently underway, although the recruitment status of this study is now listed as unknown due to an absence of reporting (https://clinicaltrials.gov/).

The Promise of STAT3 Anti-sense Oligonucleotide Inhibitors

Therapeutic nucleic acid-based approaches hold considerable potential for inhibiting a subset of the targets currently viewed as "undruggable". To date, antisense oligonucleotide (ASO) inhibitors have been tested for the treatment of a variety of diseases, including cancers. They have several advantages over pharmacological compounds: they can be designed on the basis of the gene sequence alone, and most of their associated toxicities are generally independent of the specific sequence or the molecular target, and are related to the class of compound. These effects fortunately occur at doses that are significantly higher than those that have typically been employed in trials. After promising preclinical studies in mice and monkeys, a STAT3 ASO, AZD9150 (previously known as ISIS 481464), is being evaluated in patients with lymphoma (Table 2).

AZD9150 (AstraZeneca Inc.) is a constrained ethyl modified phosphorothioate ASO that targets human *STAT3* mRNA and acts as a decoy for STAT3, but not STAT1 or STAT5. AZD9150 is highly active by free uptake in adherent and non-adherent cell-lines (including lymphoma lines), with a half-maximal inhibitory concentration (IC50) in the low nanomolar range [79]. It is well tolerated in both mice and monkeys, with little change in hematologic parameters and a transient prolongation of intrinsic clotting times [80, 81]. In the monkey, doses of 10 mg/kg body weight or greater reduced STAT3 protein levels by 90%; this is well within the range previously achieved in man using ASOs. In murine disease models using patient tumor-derived explants (PDX) or cell-line-derived xenografts, AZD9150 reduced the levels of STAT3 protein expressed within tumor cells by more than half [79], and reduced tumor volumes by about 50% in PDX models of DLBCL.

As a consequence of the anti-tumor activity observed with lymphoma cells, 12 patients with advanced lymphoma (7 with DLBCL, 2 with HL, 2 with FL, and 1 with MCL) were included in a dose escalation study, with a starting dose of 2 mg/kg [79]. The maximum tolerated dose was established as 3 mg/kg, since most patients treated at 4 mg/kg developed chronic thrombocytopenia, presumably in response to STAT3 inhibition within developing megakaryocytes. Three of six patients with treatment-refractory DLBCL showed evidence of tumor shrinkage, with two achieving a durable partial response; a fourth had a sufficiently strong PR that he became eligible for and received an autologous stem cell transplant. Trials of AZD9150 as a monotherapy, or in combination with durvalumab (MEDI4736, AstraZeneca Inc.), a human monoclonal antibody directed against programmed death ligand-1 (PDL-1), are ongoing (Table 2).

First-Generation JAK Inhibitors as Mono-therapies for the Treatment of Lymphoma

Numerous compounds with JAK inhibitory activity (sometimes referred to as "Jakanibs") have been developed, with several currently under assessment in clinical trials of patients with a blood cancer. These were primarily designed as immunomodulatory drugs, given the importance of each of the four JAK family members to both hematopoiesis and the immune system. They are all "type-I" inhibitors, which bind to the ATP-binding pocket of the JAK kinase domain in its active configuration, and thereby block transfer of the phosphoryl group to the kinase (Fig. 3).

Currently, the FDA has approved two JAK inhibitors for use in humans: tofacitinib and ruxolitinib. A third approved JAKinib, oclacitinib, is for the treatment of canine allergic dermatitis. Tofacitinib (Pfizer Inc.) has demonstrated efficacy in patients with rheumatoid arthritis, as a monotherapy or in conjunction with methotrexate [82, 83], and was approved for use in 2012. It is also being

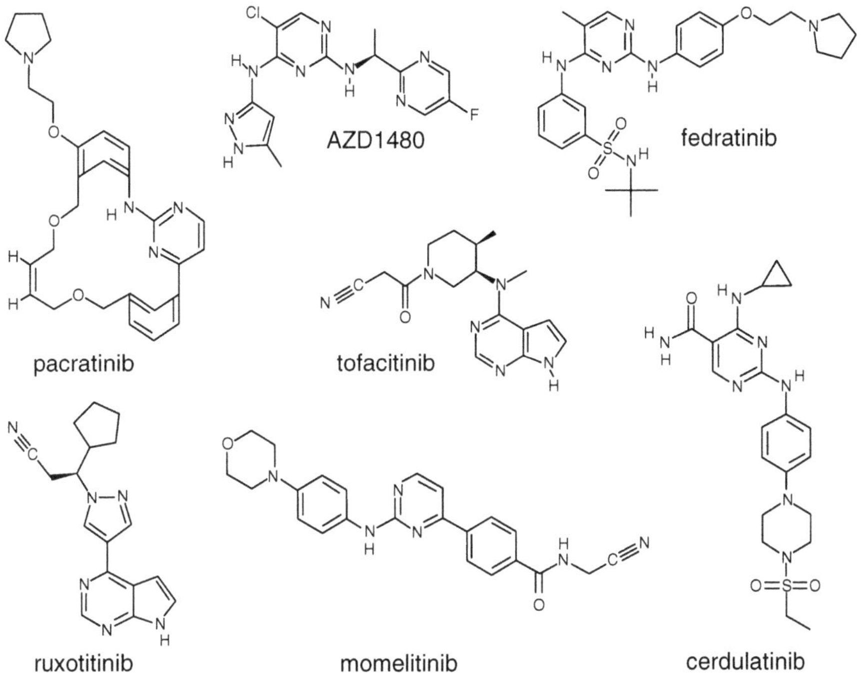

Fig. 3 *The chemical structure of JAKinibs clinically in use or being investigated.* Shown (clockwise from top left) are the structures of the JAKinibs: pacritinib, (16*E*)-11-[2-(1-Pyrrolidinyl)ethoxyl]-14,19-dioxa-5,7,26-triazatetracycl[19.3.1.1^{2,6}.1^{8,12}]heptacosa-1(25), 2 (26),3,5,8,10,12(27),16,21,23-decaene; AZD1480, 5-chloro-2-N-[(1S)-1-fluoropyrimidin-2-yl)ethyl]-4-N-(5-methyl-1H-pyrazol-3-yl)pyrimidine-2,4-diamine; fedratinib, N-*tert*-Butyl-3-{5-methyl-2-[4-(2-pyrrolidin-1-yl-ethoxy)-phenylamino]-pyrimidin-4-ylamino}astrabenzene sulfonamide; cerdulatinib, 4-(cyclopropylamino)-2-[4-(4-ethylsulfonylpiperazin-1-yl)anilino]pyrimidine-5-carboxamide; momelitinib, *N*-(cyanomethyl)-4-{2-[4-(morpholin-4-yl)aniline]pyrimidin-4-yl}benzamide; ruxolitinib, 3R)-3-cyclopentyl-3-[4-(7H-pyrrolo[2,3-d]pyrimidin-4-yl) pyrazol-1-yl]propanenitrile; and Tofacitinib, or 3-[(3R,4R)-4-methyl-3-[methyl(7H–pyrrolo[2,3-d]Pyrimidin-4-yl)amino]piperidin-1-yl]-3-oxopropanenitrile

investigated for use in other inflammatory diseases, including psoriasis and ulcerative colitis. Ruxolitinib (Novartis Pharmaceuticals) has shown particular clinical utility in treating patients with an MPN, receiving approval in 2011 for the treatment of patients with myelofibrosis, and in 2014 for patients with polycythemia vera who have had an inadequate response to, or are intolerant of, hydroxyurea. It is now being evaluated in adults with relapsed or refractory acute myeloid leukemia [84]. Topical ruxolitinib treatment is being investigated for autoimmune and inflammatory disorders, such as psoriasis [85] and alopecia areata [86]. A Phase III trial of ruxolitinib plus gemcitabine for advanced pancreatic adenocarcinoma was however terminated earlier this year due to insufficient efficacy, despite this drug combination being well tolerated and increasing overall survival over gemcitabine alone [87].

Details regarding those Jakinibs that have been evaluated in vivo, and that might show utility in treating lymphoma, are provided below; their respective chemical structures are also given in Fig. 3. Details of other promising JAK inhibitors, such as filogitinib (GLPG-0634, Galapagos NV), upadicitinib (ABT-494, AbbVie), gandotinib (LY2784544; Eli Lilly and Co.), and AC430 (Daiichi Sankyo Inc.), have not been included within this list since their evaluation in vivo remains ongoing.

Pacritinib The first Phase I trial to evaluate the safety and efficacy of a JAK inhibitor in patients with lymphoma involved pacritinib (SB1518; Cell Therapeutics Inc.). This drug is a macro-cyclic pyrimidine-based inhibitor with activity against FLT3 (with an IC50 of 23 nM) and JAK2 (with IC50 values of 23 nM for wildtype JAK2 and 19 nM for JAK2V617F). Thirty-four patients with refractory or relapsed lymphoma (HL, NHL, FL or MCL) received at least one dose of Pacritinib (ranging from 100–600 mg/day); seventeen were treated for at least 3 months, and six for 6 months. The drug had a favorable safety profile, with minimal toxicity; the most frequent adverse effects were grade II diarrhea and nausea. Thirty-one of the patients had pre- and post-baseline computed tomography (CT) scans to evaluate disease status; seventeen cases (55%) showed a decrease in tumor volume, ranging from 4–70%, following treatment with pacritinib [88].

Ruxolitinib Ruxolitinib is a pyrrolo[2,3-d]pyrimidine analog that exhibits nanomolar affinity for JAK1 and JAK2 (with IC50 values of 2.7 nM and 4.5 nM, respectively). The effects of ruxolitinib on primary lymphoma cell proliferation in vitro or in vivo have not been evaluated. However, in a multi-center study of patients with myelofibrosis, this drug was well tolerated [89]. In 2011, two randomized Phase III trials in patients with myelofibrosis were reported: COMFORT-I, a placebo-controlled trial of 309 patients; and COMFORT-II, a comparison of ruxolitinib to best available therapy involving 219 patients [90, 91]. Almost all patients treated with ruxolitinib had a reduction in spleen volume, and half reported an overall improvement in quality-of-life. The most frequent adverse events were anemia and/or thrombocytopenia; these could be managed by a dose reduction or brief interruption in treatment. Drug-mediated reductions in circulating pro-inflammatory cytokine levels were attributed to its inhibitory effects on JAK1-mediated signaling [89], a finding which suggests ruxolitinib may be an attractive therapeutic agent for lymphoma patients in which JAK1 is activated (such as those carrying a MYD88 mutation).

Pre-clinical data regarding the efficacy of ruxolitinib in treating lymphoma are rare. However, Perez and colleagues showed that exposure of cutaneous T-cell lymphoma (CTCL) cell-lines caused a dose-dependent inhibition of cell proliferation by a mechanism that impacted on the control of DNA synthesis, with a significant reduction in the basal levels of phospho-STAT3 [16]. The response of the three cell-lines tested to tofacitinib (detailed below) was similar [27], with a dose-dependent inhibition of proliferation accompanied by decreased levels of phospho-STAT3 and phospho-STAT5. These studies together suggest that lymphomagenesis may be negatively impacted in patients with CTCL by treatment with either of the Jakinibs currently approved for clinical use. Currently, there are ongoing Phase II trials evaluating ruxolitinib in the treatment of relapsed or refractory cHL, advanced HL, and relapsed DLBCL and T-cell lymphoma.

Cerdulatinib Cerdulatinib (PRT062070; Portola Pharmaceuticals) is an orally available small-molecule ATP-competitive inhibitor that inhibits the activity of SYK, JAK1, JAK2, JAK3 and TYK2 (IC50 values of 32 nM, 12 nM, 6 nM, 8 nM, and 0.5 nM, respectively) [92]. The activity of cerdulatinib has been investigated in a panel of DLBCL cell-lines (ABC and GCB subtypes); all demonstrated sensitivity to cerdulatinib with IC50 at or below 2 µM. Cerdulatinib exposure inhibited cellular metabolic function, viability, cell cycling, and signal transduction via the SYK-PLCγ2-AKT or JAK/STAT pathways [92]. It also induced cell death in primary DLBCL cells, with the degree of apoptosis correlating with the decrease in p-ERK levels. Cerdulatinib is under investigation as a monotherapy in a dose escalation study of relapsed/refractory CLL and B-cell NHL (NCT01994382), and an ongoing Phase 1/IIA trial evaluating cerdulatinib in the treatment of FL, PTCL, CTCL, and aggressive NHL.

Fedratinib Fedratinib (TG101348, SAR302503; Sanofi Aventis) has significant selectivity for JAK2 over JAK1 or JAK3 (IC50s of less than 2 nM, 132 nM, and 250 nM, respectively), and has inhibitory activity against FLT3, TRK and RET. In a Phase I study of intermediate-risk or high-risk myelofibrosis, fedratinib significantly reduced spleen volumes in 40% of patients [93]; the most frequent hematologic adverse event observed was myelosuppression. Clinical development of fedratinib was halted due to unexpected neurotoxicity. Nevertheless, pre-clinical studies with this drug provide important insights into the clinical utility of JAK inhibitors for the treatment of lymphoma [94]. Exposure of several 9p24 amplicon-positive cHL and PMBCL cell-lines to fedratinib significantly inhibited their proliferation and viability, with an inverse correlation between the IC50 of the drug and the cell-line 9p24 copy number [73, 94]. Treatment with fedratinib reduced levels of MYC and phosphorylated JAK2, STAT1, STAT3 and STAT6 in a dose-dependent manner [94]. In xenografts using 9p24 amplicon-positive cHL or PMBCL cell-lines, exposure to 120 mg/kg fedratinib for 5 days caused a significant decrease in phospho-STAT3 levels in tumor cells, and decreased their rate of growth and prolonged animal survival.

Tofacitinib Tofacitinib (CP-690550) is a small molecule JAK inhibitor that preferentially inhibits JAK1 and JAK3 signaling, but also that inhibits JAK2 and TYK2. The drug is well tolerated in patients, with a low occurrence of serious adverse effects. In a Phase II trial in patients with moderate-to-severe ulcerative colitis, tofacitinib was associated with dose-dependent improvements in response and clinical remission compared to placebo [95]. Similarly, in two Phase II trials (NCT01276639, NCT01309737) in patients with moderate-to-severe plaque psoriasis treatment was associated with a rapid reduction in psoriatic symptoms affecting the skin and nails.

Momelitinib Momelitinib (CYT-387; Gilead Sciences) is an ATP competitive inhibitor of JAK1 and JAK2, with IC50 values of 11 nM and 18 nM, respectively. A phase III clinical trial in patients with myelofibrosis ("SIMPLIFY-1", NCT01969838) was completed in June 2016; an analysis of the data obtained has not yet been published. However, one institutional report documented that 44% of patients experienced peripheral neuropathy following treatment with this drug [96], a complication also seen with exposure to fedratinib. Nevertheless, preclinical testing in human multiple myeloma cell-lines and patient primary bone marrow samples suggest that individuals with an IL6-dependent lymphoma may benefit from momelitinib treatment. In these studies, cell proliferation was inhibited in a time- and dose-dependent fashion, with reduced levels of phospho-STAT3 that were induced by IL6, cell cycle arrest, and apoptosis [97]. However, the effects of momelitinib exposure on lymphomagenesis have not been investigated.

AZD1480 AZD1480 (AstraZenca Inc.) is a pyrazol pyrimidine ATP-competitive inhibitor of JAK1 and JAK2, with respective IC50 values of 1.4 nM and 0.4 nM; at higher concentrations, it also inhibits the activities of JAK3, TYK2 and Aurora-A kinase. Treatment of HL cell-lines with varying doses of AZD1480 revealed that phosphorylated STAT1, STAT3, STAT5 and STAT6 levels were all reduced significantly at low doses (0.1–1 nM), although viability and proliferation rates were not altered [98]. At doses above 1 nM, AZD1480 induced G2/M cell cycle arrest and apoptosis, as the result of inhibition of Aurora A kinase activity. Clinical evaluation of AZD1480 in patients with lymphoma was not reported; further clinical development of this drug has been halted for unspecified reasons.

Lestaurtinib Lestauritinib (CEP-701; Cephalon Inc.) is an orally available indolocarbazole derivative originally identified as an inhibitor of the neurotropin receptor, TrkA, but found to have potent activity against FLT3 and JAK2. In Phase II trials involving patients with AML, lestauritinib it was well tolerated and induced reductions in the number of blasts present in the blood and marrow of FLT3-mutated patients [99, 100]. In patients with an MPN, however, adverse events were more common, resulting a 60% patient withdrawal rate [101, 102]. Investigators concluded that lestauritinib had only modest efficacy in patients with essential thrombocythemia or polycythemia vera (NCT00586651), or those with myelofibrosis (NCT00494585). Although lestauritinib was recently identified in a synthetic lethal screen for compounds that inhibit survival in the BCL6-deficient BL cell-line, DG75-AB7 [103], it has not yet been tested in patients with lymphoma.

Use of First-Generation JAK Inhibitors in Conjunction with Other Agents

Rather than using the afore-mentioned JAK inhibitors as monotherapies, they could be used in conjunction with existing chemotherapies, with other agents that also inhibit JAK activity, or with agents that target other functionally important intracellular signaling pathways. There are several ongoing investigations testing Jakinibs in combination with other drugs (Table 2): lestauritinib plus conventional chemotherapy for pediatric patients with AML or ALL, and ruxolitinib plus DNA methyltransferase inhibitors (such as azacytidine or decitabine), histone deacetylase inhibitors (panobinostat), or inhibitors of Hedgehog (LDE225 or PF04449913). Four ongoing clinical trials of particular interest, as they are focused on the treatment of lymphoma patients (Table 2): a study of ruxolitinib in PMBCL and relapsed or refractory HL; a dose escalation study to determine the maximum tolerated dose of ruxolitinib and bortezomib in patients with relapsed or refractory lymphoma; a combination of INCB039110, a JAK1/2 inhibitor currently being evaluated as a monotherapy for psoriasis and rheumatoid arthritis, with ibrutinib for patients with relapsed or refractory DLBCL; and INCB039110 together with INCB040093, a PI-3-Kδ inhibitor, for patients with relapsed or refractory cHL.

One promising combination therapy involves the pairing of ruxolitinib with inhibitors of heat-shock protein 90 (HSP90). HSP90 is a ubiquitously expressed protein chaperone that stabilizes a variety of different proteins, including tyrosine kinases. Pharmacologic inhibition of HSP90 in cHL cells significantly reduced cell proliferation and phospho-JAK1, -JAK2, -JAK3 and -TYK2 levels [104]. PU-H71, a purine scaffold HSP90 inhibitor, also facilitated the degradation of wildtype and mutant JAK2 in a dose-dependent fashion, improved survival in a murine model of essential thrombocythemia, and inhibited the growth of primary *JAK2V617F*-positive blood cells from patients with an MPN [105]. PU-H71 and fedratinib had additive effects in vitro, consistent with them having a shared mechanism of action. Similar findings were noted in ALL cells carrying a gain-of-function *JAK2* mutation in vitro and in PDX models [106]. Collectively, these studies provide compelling evidence for the implementation of clinical trials in patients with aberrant JAK/STAT signaling that evaluate the efficacy of a Jakinib in combination with an HSP90 inhibitor.

Resistance, Persistence, and the Development of Type-II JAK Inhibitors

Development of therapies targeted at activating kinase mutations has undoubtedly improved outcomes for patients, although acquired resistance arising from the secondary acquisition of mutations in the targeted kinase, which interfere with the inhibitory activity of the drug, is a significant issue [107–109]. JAK2 mutations have been identified that were acquired in vitro in response to continued exposure to JAK inhibitors and that confer drug resistance [106, 110–112]; several of these are located close to the ATP-binding site of the JAK2 kinase domain. Surprisingly, however, there have been no reports of secondary resistance mutations arising in MPN patients treated with ruxolitinib. As the presence of these mutations could be considered an indicator of an effective therapy, with sufficient targeting achieved to select for genetic resistance, an absence may suggest that the limited therapeutic efficacy of ruxolitinib in patients is due to insufficient JAK inhibition.

Despite chronic exposure to ruxolitinib in vitro, a proportion of *JAK2V617F*-positive cells survive without having acquired secondary resistance mutations [106, 113], with a 12-fold increase in IC50 compared to parental cells [114]. These cells, and ones arising in the presence of tofacitinib and other Jakinibs, were characterized by increased JAK2 activation loop phosphorylation. Biochemical studies revealed that cells had instead acquired an adaptive form of resistance in which JAK2 was stabilized by binding to a type I JAK inhibitor [113, 115], which facilitated the heterodimeric association of JAK2 with JAK1 or TYK2, resulting in the phosphorylation of JAK2 residues Y1007/1008, and reactivation of JAK/STAT signaling. The exact nature of the mechanism responsible for this resistance, which has been termed "persistence", is currently unclear. Persistence is not solely an in vitro phenomenon; it was also noted in a murine model of essential thrombocythemia in which bone marrow cells express mutant MPL [116], and in the granulocytes of MPN patients treated with ruxolitinib, but not those from drug-naive patients. Importantly, in vitro persistence was reversible, with the removal of ruxolitinib from cell cultures for 2–4 weeks resensitizing them to this and other Jakinibs. Knockdown of JAK1 and TYK2 in vitro similarly increased the sensitivity of persistent cells to ruxolitinib but had little effect on parental cells, whereas the knockdown of JAK2 caused growth suppression and the loss of downstream signaling events [113]. Taken together, the data suggested that patients receiving ruxolitinib might benefit from periodic interruptions to their treatment, or from combination therapies in which either JAK2 activity is concurrently targeted by a different approach (such as use of an HSP90 inhibitor), or the activity of JAK1 and TYK2 is simultaneously reduced.

Whereas type I kinase inhibitors bind their targets in the kinase-active conformation, the type II inhibitors engage them in the inactive conformation. The dihydroindole, NVP-BBT594, was found to bind to wildtype and mutant JAK2 in the inactive confirmation, and to suppress activation loop phosphorylation, and STAT phosphorylation [115]. These findings prompted the development of NVP-CHZ868, another type II inhibitor, which has activity against JAK2 and TYK2, but not JAK1 or JAK3 [117]. Biochemical studies revealed that CHZ868 stabilizes and locks JAK2 in an inactive conformation. In BaF3 cells expressing the ALL-associated JAK2R683G mutant, treatment with type I inhibitors induced JAK2 hyper-phosphorylation, whereas CHZ868 abrogated levels of phospho-JAK2 and phospho-STAT5. CHZ868 was also 40-times more potent than type I inhibitors in an ALL-derived cell-line carrying a *CRLF2* rearrangement and JAK2I682F mutation. CHZ868 was well tolerated in mice, with no perturbations in hematopoiesis noted in animals treated daily for

3–6 weeks at a dose of 30 mg/kg body weight. Mice engrafted with three different *CRLF2*-rearranged PDXs showed reduced splenomegaly and lower white cell counts in the peripheral blood following 6 days treatment with CHZ868, and had improved overall survival rates compared to controls [117]. In a murine model of *JAK2V617F*-positive polycythemia vera, CHZ868 normalized spleen and liver weights, and restored the hematocrit to normal levels [114]. Similarly, in a model of *MPLW515L*-associated myelofibrosis, treatment normalized spleen sizes, reduced leukocytosis and hepatomegaly in a dose-dependent manner, decreased reticulin fiber deposition within the marrow and spleen, and prolonged survival [114]. Importantly, in both disease models, the proportion of mutation-positive cells present was reduced by exposure to drug, suggesting that alternative approaches to JAK2 inhibition, including the use of type II inhibitors, may increase the therapeutic benefit to patients.

Future Directions

Although the first JAK inhibitor for use in humans was approved only 5 years ago, the development of next-generation inhibitors that promise to more efficiently target and inhibit deregulated JAK/STAT signaling in blood cells has already begun. Additional advances are likely once the biological activity of the four JAK family members is more fully appreciated, particularly with regards to the role of the pseudokinase domain on JAK regulation, since it is the site of the majority of activating JAK mutations in lymphoma and in other blood cancers. Similarly, the development of antisense oligonucleotides to inhibit individual STAT family members might enable the activities of these once "undruggable" targets to be normalized in patients with a blood cancer.

References

1. Saharinen P, Takaluoma K, Silvennoinen O. Regulation of the Jak2 tyrosine kinase by its pseudokinase domain. Mol Cell Biol. 2000;20(10):3387–95.
2. Saharinen P, Silvennoinen O. The pseudokinase domain is required for suppression of basal activity of Jak2 and Jak3 tyrosine kinases and for cytokine-inducible activation of signal transduction. J Biol Chem. 2002;277(49):47954–63.
3. Brooks AJ, Dai W, O'Mara ML, Abankwa D, Chhabra Y, Pelekanos RA, et al. Mechanism of activation of protein kinase JAK2 by the growth hormone receptor. Science. 2014;344(6185):1249783.
4. Rinaldi CR, Rinaldi P, Alagia A, Gemei M, Esposito N, Formiggini F, et al. Preferential nuclear accumulation of JAK2V617F in CD34+ but not in granulocytic, megakaryocytic, or erythroid cells of patients with Philadelphia-negative myeloproliferative neoplasia. Blood. 2010;116(26):6023–6.
5. Dawson MA, Bannister AJ, Gottgens B, Foster SD, Bartke T, Green AR, et al. JAK2 phosphorylates histone H3Y41 and excludes HP1alpha from chromatin. Nature. 2009;461(7265):819–22.

6. Griffiths DS, Li J, Dawson MA, Trotter MW, Cheng YH, Smith AM, et al. LIF-independent JAK signalling to chromatin in embryonic stem cells uncovered from an adult stem cell disease. Nat Cell Biol. 2011;13(1):13–21.
7. Dawson MA, Foster SD, Bannister AJ, Robson SC, Hannah R, Wang X, et al. Three distinct patterns of histone H3Y41 phosphorylation mark active genes. Cell Rep. 2012;2(3):470–7.
8. Pollack BP, Kotenko SV, He W, Izotova LS, Barnoski BL, Pestka S. The human homologue of the yeast proteins Skb1 and Hsl7p interacts with Jak kinases and contains protein methyltransferase activity. J Biol Chem. 1999;274(44):31531–42.
9. Liu F, Zhao X, Perna F, Wang L, Koppikar P, Abdel-Wahab O, et al. JAK2V617F-mediated phosphorylation of PRMT5 downregulates its methyltransferase activity and promotes myeloproliferation. Cancer Cell. 2011;19(2):283–94.
10. Sahasrabuddhe AA, Chen X, Chung F, Velusamy T, Lim MS, Elenitoba-Johnson KS. Oncogenic Y641 mutations in EZH2 prevent Jak2/beta-TrCP-mediated degradation. Oncogene. 2015;34(4):445–54.
11. Kuzmichev A, Nishioka K, Erdjument-Bromage H, Tempst P, Reinberg D. Histone methyltransferase activity associated with a human multiprotein complex containing the Enhancer of Zeste protein. Genes Dev. 2002;16(22):2893–905.
12. Cao R, Wang L, Wang H, Xia L, Erdjument-Bromage H, Tempst P, et al. Role of histone H3 lysine 27 methylation in Polycomb-group silencing. Science. 2002;298(5595):1039–43.
13. Rosenwald A, Wright G, Leroy K, Yu X, Gaulard P, Gascoyne RD, et al. Molecular diagnosis of primary mediastinal B cell lymphoma identifies a clinically favorable subgroup of diffuse large B cell lymphoma related to Hodgkin lymphoma. J Exp Med. 2003;198(6):851–62.
14. Savage KJ, Monti S, Kutok JL, Cattoretti G, Neuberg D, De Leval L, et al. The molecular signature of mediastinal large B-cell lymphoma differs from that of other diffuse large B-cell lymphomas and shares features with classical Hodgkin lymphoma. Blood. 2003;102(12):3871–9.
15. Roberti A, Dobay MP, Bisig B, Vallois D, Boechat C, Lanitis E, et al. Type II enteropathy-associated T-cell lymphoma features a unique genomic profile with highly recurrent SETD2 alterations. Nat Comm. 2016;7:12602.
16. Perez C, Gonzalez-Rincon J, Onaindia A, Almaraz C, Garcia-Diaz N, Pisonero H, et al. Mutated JAK kinases and deregulated STAT activity are potential therapeutic targets in cutaneous T-cell lymphoma. Haematologica. 2015;100(11):e450–3.
17. Crescenzo R, Abate F, Lasorsa E, Tabbo F, Gaudiano M, Chiesa N, et al. Convergent mutations and kinase fusions lead to oncogenic STAT3 activation in anaplastic large cell lymphoma. Cancer Cell. 2015;27(4):516–32.
18. Joos S, Otano-Joos MI, Ziegler S, Bruderlein S, du Manoir S, Bentz M, et al. Primary mediastinal (thymic) B-cell lymphoma is characterized by gains of chromosomal material including 9p and amplification of the REL gene. Blood. 1996;87(4):1571–8.
19. Green MR, Monti S, Rodig SJ, Juszczynski P, Currie T, O'Donnell E, et al. Integrative analysis reveals selective 9p24.1 amplification, increased PD-1 ligand expression, and further induction via JAK2 in nodular sclerosing Hodgkin lymphoma and primary mediastinal large B-cell lymphoma. Blood. 2010;116(17):3268–77.
20. Eberle FC, Salaverria I, Steidl C, Summers TA Jr, Pittaluga S, Neriah SB, et al. Gray zone lymphoma: chromosomal aberrations with immunophenotypic and clinical correlations. Mod Pathol. 2011;24(12):1586–97.
21. Joos S, Kupper M, Ohl S, von Bonin F, Mechtersheimer G, Bentz M, et al. Genomic imbalances including amplification of the tyrosine kinase gene JAK2 in CD30+ Hodgkin cells. Cancer Res. 2000;60(3):549–52.
22. Roncero AM, Lopez-Nieva P, Cobos-Fernandez MA, Villa-Morales M, Gonzalez-Sanchez L, Lopez-Lorenzo JL, et al. Contribution of JAK2 mutations to T-cell lymphoblastic lymphoma development. Leukemia. 2016;30(1):94–103.

23. Nairismagi ML, Tan J, Lim JQ, Nagarajan S, Ng CC, Rajasegaran V, et al. JAK-STAT and G-protein-coupled receptor signaling pathways are frequently altered in epitheliotropic intestinal T-cell lymphoma. Leukemia. 2016;30(6):1311–9.
24. Bouchekioua A, Scourzic L, de Wever O, Zhang Y, Cervera P, Aline-Fardin A, et al. JAK3 deregulation by activating mutations confers invasive growth advantage in extranodal nasal-type natural killer cell lymphoma. Leukemia. 2014;28(2):338–48.
25. Koo GC, Tan SY, Tang T, Poon SL, Allen GE, Tan L, et al. Janus kinase 3-activating mutations identified in natural killer/T-cell lymphoma. Cancer Dis. 2012;2(7):591–7.
26. Elliott NE, Cleveland SM, Grann V, Janik J, Waldmann TA, Dave UP. FERM domain mutations induce gain of function in JAK3 in adult T-cell leukemia/lymphoma. Blood. 2011;118(14):3911–21.
27. McGirt LY, Jia P, Baerenwald DA, Duszynski RJ, Dahlman KB, Zic JA, et al. Whole-genome sequencing reveals oncogenic mutations in mycosis fungoides. Blood. 2015;126(4):508–19.
28. da Silva Almeida AC, Abate F, Khiabanian H, Martinez-Escala E, Guitart J, Tensen CP, et al. The mutational landscape of cutaneous T cell lymphoma and Sezary syndrome. Nat Genet. 2015;47(12):1465–70.
29. Cornejo MG, Kharas MG, Werneck MB, Le Bras S, Moore SA, Ball B, et al. Constitutive JAK3 activation induces lymphoproliferative syndromes in murine bone marrow transplantation models. Blood. 2009;113(12):2746–54.
30. Woollard WJ, Pullabhatla V, Lorenc A, Patel VM, Butler RM, Bayega A, et al. Candidate driver genes involved in genome maintenance and DNA repair in Sezary syndrome. Blood. 2016;127(26):3387–97.
31. Couronne L, Scourzic L, Pilati C, Valle VD, Duffourd Y, Solary E, et al. STAT3 mutations identified in human hematologic neoplasms induce myeloid malignancies in a mouse bone marrow transplantation model. Haematologica. 2013;98(11):1748–52.
32. Kucuk C, Jiang B, Hu X, Zhang W, Chan JK, Xiao W, et al. Activating mutations of STAT5B and STAT3 in lymphomas derived from gammadelta-T or NK cells. Nat Comm. 2015;6:6025.
33. Jiang L, Gu ZH, Yan ZX, Zhao X, Xie YY, Zhang ZG, et al. Exome sequencing identifies somatic mutations of DDX3X in natural killer/T-cell lymphoma. Nat Genet. 2015;47(9):1061–6.
34. Ritz O, Guiter C, Castellano F, Dorsch K, Melzner J, Jais JP, et al. Recurrent mutations of the STAT6 DNA binding domain in primary mediastinal B-cell lymphoma. Blood. 2009;114(6):1236–42.
35. Morin RD, Assouline S, Alcaide M, Mohajeri A, Johnston RL, Chong L, et al. Genetic landscapes of relapsed and refractory diffuse large B-cell lymphomas. Clin Cancer Res. 2016;22(9):2290–300.
36. Yildiz M, Li H, Bernard D, Amin NA, Ouilette P, Jones S, et al. Activating STAT6 mutations in follicular lymphoma. Blood. 2015;125(4):668–79.
37. Gunawardana J, Chan FC, Telenius A, Woolcock B, Kridel R, Tan KL, et al. Recurrent somatic mutations of PTPN1 in primary mediastinal B cell lymphoma and Hodgkin lymphoma. Nat Genet. 2014;46(4):329–35.
38. Kleppe M, Tousseyn T, Geissinger E, Kalender Atak Z, Aerts S, Rosenwald A, et al. Mutation analysis of the tyrosine phosphatase PTPN2 in Hodgkin's lymphoma and T-cell non-Hodgkin's lymphoma. Haematologica. 2011;96(11):1723–7.
39. Demosthenous C, Han JJ, Hu G, Stenson M, Gupta M. Loss of function mutations in PTPN6 promote STAT3 deregulation via JAK3 kinase in diffuse large B-cell lymphoma. Oncotarget. 2015;6(42):44703–13.
40. Weniger MA, Melzner I, Menz CK, Wegener S, Bucur AJ, Dorsch K, et al. Mutations of the tumor suppressor gene SOCS-1 in classical Hodgkin lymphoma are frequent and associated with nuclear phospho-STAT5 accumulation. Oncogene. 2006;25(18):2679–84.
41. Lennerz JK, Hoffmann K, Bubolz AM, Lessel D, Welke C, Ruther N, et al. Suppressor of cytokine signaling 1 gene mutation status as a prognostic biomarker in classical Hodgkin lymphoma. Oncotarget. 2015;6(30):29097–110.

42. Mottok A, Renne C, Seifert M, Oppermann E, Bechstein W, Hansmann ML, et al. Inactivating SOCS1 mutations are caused by aberrant somatic hypermutation and restricted to a subset of B-cell lymphoma entities. Blood. 2009;114(20):4503–6.
43. Schif B, Lennerz JK, Kohler CW, Bentink S, Kreuz M, Melzner I, et al. SOCS1 mutation subtypes predict divergent outcomes in diffuse large B-cell lymphoma (DLBCL) patients. Oncotarget. 2013;4(1):35–47.
44. Lenz G, Wright GW, Emre NC, Kohlhammer H, Dave SS, Davis RE, et al. Molecular subtypes of diffuse large B-cell lymphoma arise by distinct genetic pathways. Proc Natl Acad Sci U S A. 2008;105(36):13520–5.
45. Meier C, Hoeller S, Bourgau C, Hirschmann P, Schwaller J, Went P, et al. Recurrent numerical aberrations of JAK2 and deregulation of the JAK2-STAT cascade in lymphomas. Mod Pathol. 2009;22(3):476–87.
46. Rui L, Emre NC, Kruhlak MJ, Chung HJ, Steidl C, Slack G, et al. Cooperative epigenetic modulation by cancer amplicon genes. Cancer Cell. 2010;18(6):590–605.
47. Cloos PA, Christensen J, Agger K, Maiolica A, Rappsilber J, Antal T, et al. The putative oncogene GASC1 demethylates tri- and dimethylated lysine 9 on histone H3. Nature. 2006;442(7100):307–11.
48. Blombery P, Thompson ER, Jones K, Arnau GM, Lade S, Markham JF, et al. Whole exome sequencing reveals activating JAK1 and STAT3 mutations in breast implant-associated anaplastic large cell lymphoma anaplastic large cell lymphoma. Haematologica. 2016;101(9):e387–90.
49. Staerk J, Kallin A, Demoulin JB, Vainchenker W, Constantinescu SN. JAK1 and Tyk2 activation by the homologous polycythemia vera JAK2 V617F mutation: cross-talk with IGF1 receptor. J Biol Chem. 2005;280(51):41893–9.
50. Baxter EJ, Scott LM, Campbell PJ, East C, Fourouclas N, Swanton S, et al. Acquired mutation of the tyrosine kinase JAK2 in human myeloproliferative disorders. Lancet. 2005;365(9464):1054–61.
51. Levine RL, Wadleigh M, Cools J, Ebert BL, Wernig G, Huntly BJ, et al. Activating mutation in the tyrosine kinase JAK2 in polycythemia vera, essential thrombocythemia, and myeloid metaplasia with myelofibrosis. Cancer Cell. 2005;7(4):387–97.
52. Kralovics R, Passamonti F, Buser AS, Teo SS, Tiedt R, Passweg JR, et al. A gain-of-function mutation of JAK2 in myeloproliferative disorders. N Engl J Med. 2005;352(17):1779–90.
53. James C, Ugo V, Le Couedic JP, Staerk J, Delhommeau F, Lacout C, et al. A unique clonal JAK2 mutation leading to constitutive signalling causes polycythaemia vera. Nature. 2005;434(7037):1144–8.
54. Scott LM, Tong W, Levine RL, Scott MA, Beer PA, Stratton MR, et al. JAK2 exon 12 mutations in polycythemia vera and idiopathic erythrocytosis. N Engl J Med. 2007;356(5):459–68.
55. Bercovich D, Ganmore I, Scott LM, Wainreb G, Birger Y, Elimelech A, et al. Mutations of JAK2 in acute lymphoblastic leukaemias associated with Down's syndrome. Lancet. 2008;372(9648):1484–92.
56. Mullighan CG, Zhang J, Harvey RC, Collins-Underwood JR, Schulman BA, Phillips LA, et al. JAK mutations in high-risk childhood acute lymphoblastic leukemia. Proc Natl Acad Sci U S A. 2009;106(23):9414–8.
57. Scott LM, Campbell PJ, Baxter EJ, Todd T, Stephens P, Edkins S, et al. The V617F JAK2 mutation is uncommon in cancers and in myeloid malignancies other than the classic myeloproliferative disorders. Blood. 2005;106(8):2920–1.
58. Melzner I, Weniger MA, Menz CK, Moller P. Absence of the JAK2 V617F activating mutation in classical Hodgkin lymphoma and primary mediastinal B-cell lymphoma. Leukemia. 2006;20(1):157–8.
59. Wu D, Dutra B, Lindeman N, Takahashi H, Takeyama K, Harris NL, et al. No evidence for the JAK2 (V617F) or JAK2 exon 12 mutations in primary mediastinal large B-cell lymphoma. Diagn Mol Pathol. 2009;18(3):144–9.

60. Van Roosbroeck K, Cox L, Tousseyn T, Lahortiga I, Gielen O, Cauwelier B, et al. JAK2 rearrangements, including the novel SEC31A-JAK2 fusion, are recurrent in classical Hodgkin lymphoma. Blood. 2011;117(15):4056–64.
61. Walters DK, Mercher T, Gu TL, O'Hare T, Tyner JW, Loriaux M, et al. Activating alleles of JAK3 in acute megakaryoblastic leukemia. Cancer Cell. 2006;10(1):65–75.
62. Morin RD, Mendez-Lago M, Mungall AJ, Goya R, Mungall KL, Corbett RD, et al. Frequent mutation of histone-modifying genes in non-Hodgkin lymphoma. Nature. 2011;476(7360):298–303.
63. Lohr JG, Stojanov P, Lawrence MS, Auclair D, Chapuy B, Sougnez C, et al. Discovery and prioritization of somatic mutations in diffuse large B-cell lymphoma (DLBCL) by whole-exome sequencing. Proc Natl Acad Sci U S A. 2012;109(10):3879–84.
64. Koskela HL, Eldfors S, Ellonen P, van Adrichem AJ, Kuusanmaki H, Andersson EI, et al. Somatic STAT3 mutations in large granular lymphocytic leukemia. N Engl J Med. 2012;366(20):1905–13.
65. Hu G, Witzig TE, Gupta M. A novel missense (M206K) STAT3 mutation in diffuse large B cell lymphoma deregulates STAT3 signaling. PLoS One. 2013;8(7):e67851.
66. Okosun J, Bodor C, Wang J, Araf S, Yang CY, Pan C, et al. Integrated genomic analysis identifies recurrent mutations and evolution patterns driving the initiation and progression of follicular lymphoma. Nat Genet. 2014;46(2):176–81.
67. Mottok A, Renne C, Willenbrock K, Hansmann ML, Brauninger A. Somatic hypermutation of SOCS1 in lymphocyte-predominant Hodgkin lymphoma is accompanied by high JAK2 expression and activation of STAT6. Blood. 2007;110(9):3387–90.
68. Melzner I, Bucur AJ, Bruderlein S, Dorsch K, Hasel C, Barth TF, et al. Biallelic mutation of SOCS-1 impairs JAK2 degradation and sustains phospho-JAK2 action in the MedB-1 mediastinal lymphoma line. Blood. 2005;105(6):2535–42.
69. Chim CS, Fung TK, Cheung WC, Liang R, Kwong YL. SOCS1 and SHP1 hypermethylation in multiple myeloma: implications for epigenetic activation of the Jak/STAT pathway. Blood. 2004;103(12):4630–5.
70. Witzig TE, Hu G, Offer SM, Wellik LE, Han JJ, Stenson MJ, et al. Epigenetic mechanisms of protein tyrosine phosphatase 6 suppression in diffuse large B-cell lymphoma: implications for epigenetic therapy. Leukemia. 2014;28(1):147–54.
71. Treon SP, Xu L, Yang G, Zhou Y, Liu X, Cao Y, et al. MYD88 L265P somatic mutation in Waldenstrom's macroglobulinemia. N Engl J Med. 2012;367(9):826–33.
72. Ngo VN, Young RM, Schmitz R, Jhavar S, Xiao W, Lim KH, et al. Oncogenically active MYD88 mutations in human lymphoma. Nature. 2011;470(7332):115–9.
73. Gupta M, Han JJ, Stenson M, Maurer M, Wellik L, Hu G, et al. Elevated serum IL-10 levels in diffuse large B-cell lymphoma: a mechanism of aberrant JAK2 activation. Blood. 2012;119(12):2844–53.
74. Boi M, Gaudio E, Bonetti P, Kwee I, Bernasconi E, Tarantelli C, et al. The BET bromodomain inhibitor OTX015 affects pathogenetic pathways in preclinical B-cell tumor models and synergizes with targeted drugs. Clin Cancer Res. 2015;21(7):1628–38.
75. Ortega-Molina A, Boss IW, Canela A, Pan H, Jiang Y, Zhao C, et al. The histone lysine methyltransferase KMT2D sustains a gene expression program that represses B cell lymphoma development. Nat Med. 2015;21(10):1199–208.
76. Pasqualucci L, Dominguez-Sola D, Chiarenza A, Fabbri G, Grunn A, Trifonov V, et al. Inactivating mutations of acetyltransferase genes in B-cell lymphoma. Nature. 2011;471(7337):189–95.
77. Spina V, Khiabanian H, Messina M, Monti S, Cascione L, Bruscaggin A, et al. The genetics of nodal marginal zone lymphoma. Blood. 2016;128(10):1362–73.
78. Hayakawa F, Sugimoto K, Harada Y, Hashimoto N, Ohi N, Kurahashi S, et al. A novel STAT inhibitor, OPB-31121, has a significant antitumor effect on leukemia with STAT-addictive oncokinases. Blood Cancer J. 2013;3:e166.

79. Hong D, Kurzrock R, Kim Y, Woessner R, Younes A, Nemunaitis J, et al. AZD9150, a next-generation antisense oligonucleotide inhibitor of STAT3 with early evidence of clinical activity in lymphoma and lung cancer. Sci Transl Med. 2015;7(314):314ra185.
80. Burel SA, Han SR, Lee HS, Norris DA, Lee BS, Machemer T, et al. Preclinical evaluation of the toxicological effects of a novel constrained ethyl modified antisense compound targeting signal transducer and activator of transcription 3 in mice and cynomolgus monkeys. Nucleic Acid Ther. 2013;23(3):213–27.
81. Sen M, Paul K, Freilino ML, Li H, Li C, Johnson DE, et al. Systemic administration of a cyclic signal transducer and activator of transcription 3 (STAT3) decoy oligonucleotide inhibits tumor growth without inducing toxicological effects. Mol Med. 2014;20:46–56.
82. Fleischmann R, Kremer J, Cush J, Schulze-Koops H, Connell CA, Bradley JD, et al. Placebo-controlled trial of tofacitinib monotherapy in rheumatoid arthritis. N Engl J Med. 2012;367(6):495–507.
83. van Vollenhoven RF, Fleischmann R, Cohen S, Lee EB, Garcia Meijide JA, Wagner S, et al. Tofacitinib or adalimumab versus placebo in rheumatoid arthritis. N Engl J Med. 2012;367(6):508–19.
84. Pemmaraju N, Kantarjian H, Kadia T, Cortes J, Borthakur G, Newberry K, et al. A phase I/II study of the Janus kinase (JAK)1 and 2 inhibitor ruxolitinib in patients with relapsed or refractory acute myeloid leukemia. Clin Lymphoma Myeloma Leukemia. 2015;15(3):171–6.
85. Punwani N, Burn T, Scherle P, Flores R, Shi J, Collier P, et al. Downmodulation of key inflammatory cell markers with a topical Janus kinase 1/2 inhibitor. Br J Dermatol. 2015;173(4):989–97.
86. Xing L, Dai Z, Jabbari A, Cerise JE, Higgins CA, Gong W, et al. Alopecia areata is driven by cytotoxic T lymphocytes and is reversed by JAK inhibition. Nat Med. 2014;20(9):1043–9.
87. Hurwitz HI, Uppal N, Wagner SA, Bendell JC, Beck JT, Wade SM 3rd, et al. Randomized, double-blind, phase II study of ruxolitinib or placebo in combination with capecitabine in patients with metastatic pancreatic cancer for whom therapy with gemcitabine has failed. J Clin Oncol. 2015;33(34):4039–47.
88. Younes A, Romaguera J, Fanale M, McLaughlin P, Hagemeister F, Copeland A, et al. Phase I study of a novel oral Janus kinase 2 inhibitor, SB1518, in patients with relapsed lymphoma: evidence of clinical and biologic activity in multiple lymphoma subtypes. J Clin Oncol. 2012;30(33):4161–7.
89. Verstovsek S, Kantarjian H, Mesa RA, Pardanani AD, Cortes-Franco J, Thomas DA, et al. Safety and efficacy of INCB018424, a JAK1 and JAK2 inhibitor, in myelofibrosis. N Engl J Med. 2010;363(12):1117–27.
90. Verstovsek S, Mesa RA, Gotlib J, Levy RS, Gupta V, DiPersio JF, et al. A double-blind, placebo-controlled trial of ruxolitinib for myelofibrosis. N Engl J Med. 2012;366(9):799–807.
91. Harrison C, Kiladjian JJ, Al-Ali HK, Gisslinger H, Waltzman R, Stalbovskaya V, et al. JAK inhibition with ruxolitinib versus best available therapy for myelofibrosis. N Engl J Med. 2012;366(9):787–98.
92. Ma J, Xing W, Coffey G, Dresser K, Lu K, Guo A, et al. Cerdulatinib, a novel dual SYK/JAK kinase inhibitor, has broad anti-tumor activity in both ABC and GCB types of diffuse large B cell lymphoma. Oncotarget. 2015;6(41):43881–96.
93. Pardanani A, Gotlib JR, Jamieson C, Cortes JE, Talpaz M, Stone RM, et al. Safety and efficacy of TG101348, a selective JAK2 inhibitor, in myelofibrosis. J Clin Oncol. 2011;29(7):789–96.
94. Hao Y, Chapuy B, Monti S, Sun HH, Rodig SJ, Shipp MA. Selective JAK2 inhibition specifically decreases Hodgkin lymphoma and mediastinal large B-cell lymphoma growth in vitro and in vivo. Clin Cancer Res. 2014;20(10):2674–83.
95. Sandborn WJ, Ghosh S, Panes J, Vranic I, Su C, Rousell S, et al. Tofacitinib, an oral Janus kinase inhibitor, in active ulcerative colitis. N Engl J Med. 2012;367(7):616–24.
96. Abdelrahman RA, Begna KH, Al-Kali A, Hogan WJ, Litzow MR, Pardanani A, et al. Momelotinib treatment-emergent neuropathy: prevalence, risk factors and outcome in 100 patients with myelofibrosis. Br J Haematol. 2015;169(1):77–80.

97. Monaghan KA, Khong T, Burns CJ, Spencer A. The novel JAK inhibitor CYT387 suppresses multiple signalling pathways, prevents proliferation and induces apoptosis in phenotypically diverse myeloma cells. Leukemia. 2011;25(12):1891–9.
98. Derenzini E, Lemoine M, Buglio D, Katayama H, Ji Y, Davis RE, et al. The JAK inhibitor AZD1480 regulates proliferation and immunity in Hodgkin lymphoma. Blood Cancer J. 2011;1(12):e46.
99. Levis M, Allebach J, Tse KF, Zheng R, Baldwin BR, Smith BD, et al. A FLT3-targeted tyrosine kinase inhibitor is cytotoxic to leukemia cells in vitro and in vivo. Blood. 2002;99(11):3885–91.
100. Smith BD, Levis M, Beran M, Giles F, Kantarjian H, Berg K, et al. Single-agent CEP-701, a novel FLT3 inhibitor, shows biologic and clinical activity in patients with relapsed or refractory acute myeloid leukemia. Blood. 2004;103(10):3669–76.
101. Hexner E, Roboz G, Hoffman R, Luger S, Mascarenhas J, Carroll M, et al. Open-label study of oral CEP-701 (lestaurtinib) in patients with polycythaemia vera or essential thrombocythaemia with JAK2-V617F mutation. Br J Haematol. 2014;164(1):83–93.
102. Santos FP, Kantarjian HM, Jain N, Manshouri T, Thomas DA, Garcia-Manero G, et al. Phase 2 study of CEP-701, an orally available JAK2 inhibitor, in patients with primary or post-polycythemia vera/essential thrombocythemia myelofibrosis. Blood. 2010;115(6):1131–6.
103. Beck D, Zobel J, Barber R, Evans S, Lezina L, Allchin RL, et al. Synthetic lethal screen demonstrates that a JAK2 inhibitor suppresses a BCL6-dependent IL10RA/JAK2/STAT3 pathway in high grade B-cell lymphoma. J Biol Chem. 2016;291(32):16686–98.
104. Schoof N, von Bonin F, Trumper L, Kube D. HSP90 is essential for Jak-STAT signaling in classical Hodgkin lymphoma cells. Cell Commun Signal. 2009;7:17.
105. Marubayashi S, Koppikar P, Taldone T, Abdel-Wahab O, West N, Bhagwat N, et al. HSP90 is a therapeutic target in JAK2-dependent myeloproliferative neoplasms in mice and humans. J Clin Invest. 2010;120(10):3578–93.
106. Weigert O, Lane AA, Bird L, Kopp N, Chapuy B, van Bodegom D, et al. Genetic resistance to JAK2 enzymatic inhibitors is overcome by HSP90 inhibition. J Exp Med. 2012;209(2):259–73.
107. Engelman JA, Zejnullahu K, Mitsudomi T, Song Y, Hyland C, Park JO, et al. MET amplification leads to gefitinib resistance in lung cancer by activating ERBB3 signaling. Science. 2007;316(5827):1039–43.
108. Smith CC, Wang Q, Chin CS, Salerno S, Damon LE, Levis MJ, et al. Validation of ITD mutations in FLT3 as a therapeutic target in human acute myeloid leukaemia. Nature. 2012;485(7397):260–3.
109. Gorre ME, Mohammed M, Ellwood K, Hsu N, Paquette R, Rao PN, et al. Clinical resistance to STI-571 cancer therapy caused by BCR-ABL gene mutation or amplification. Science. 2001;293(5531):876–80.
110. Deshpande A, Reddy MM, Schade GO, Ray A, Chowdary TK, Griffin JD, et al. Kinase domain mutations confer resistance to novel inhibitors targeting JAK2V617F in myeloproliferative neoplasms. Leukemia. 2012;26(4):708–15.
111. Marit MR, Chohan M, Matthew N, Huang K, Kuntz DA, Rose DR, et al. Random mutagenesis reveals residues of JAK2 critical in evading inhibition by a tyrosine kinase inhibitor. PLoS One. 2012;7(8):e43437.
112. Hornakova T, Springuel L, Devreux J, Dusa A, Constantinescu SN, Knoops L, et al. Oncogenic JAK1 and JAK2-activating mutations resistant to ATP-competitive inhibitors. Haematologica. 2011;96(6):845–53.
113. Koppikar P, Bhagwat N, Kilpivaara O, Manshouri T, Adli M, Hricik T, et al. Heterodimeric JAK-STAT activation as a mechanism of persistence to JAK2 inhibitor therapy. Nature. 2012;489(7414):155–9.
114. Meyer SC, Keller MD, Chiu S, Koppikar P, Guryanova OA, Rapaport F, et al. CHZ868, a type II JAK2 inhibitor, reverses type I JAK inhibitor persistence and demonstrates efficacy in myeloproliferative neoplasms. Cancer Cell. 2015;28(1):15–28.

115. Andraos R, Qian Z, Bonenfant D, Rubert J, Vangrevelinghe E, Scheufler C, et al. Modulation of activation-loop phosphorylation by JAK inhibitors is binding mode dependent. Cancer Dis. 2012;2(6):512–23.
116. Pikman Y, Lee BH, Mercher T, McDowell E, Ebert BL, Gozo M, et al. MPLW515L is a novel somatic activating mutation in myelofibrosis with myeloid metaplasia. PLoS Med. 2006;3(7):e270.
117. Wu SC, Li LS, Kopp N, Montero J, Chapuy B, Yoda A, et al. Activity of the type II JAK2 inhibitor CHZ868 in B cell acute lymphoblastic leukemia. Cancer Cell. 2015;28(1):29–41.

Index

A
Acalabrutinib drug, 17
Activated B-cell DLBCL (ABC-DLBCL), 94
Activating transcription factor 6 (ATF6), 50
Alternative proliferation pathways, 94
Anaplastic large cell lymphoma (ALCL), 112
Apoptosis
  BAK/BAX with mitochrondrial disruption, 28
  BH3-proteins, 27
  intrinsic pathway, 25, 26
  venetoclax-induced, 38
Ataxia Telangiectasia Mutated (ATM) protein, 93
ATP-binding cassette B1 (ABCB1), 52
Autophosphorylation, 50, 51, 61
Azacitidine, 34
AZD1480 (AstraZenca Inc.), 124
AZD9150 (AstraZenca Inc.), 120

B
B cell lymphoma 2 (BCL2) inhibitors, 30
  ABT-737, 28
  BH3 mimetics, 28
  cancer, 26, 27
  CLL, 25, 38
  ibrutinib, 38
  intracellular cancer pathways, 38
  navitoclax, 28–30
  NHL, 25
  patients, 25
  targeted agents, 25
  venetoclax (*see* Venetoclax)
B cell receptor (BcR) signaling, 2
BcR signaling pathways, 4

BGB-3111 inhibitor, 18
Bortezomib resistance, 48, 51, 60, 62
  BCL-2 inhibition, 62
  differentiation induction, 59, 60
  immature plasma cells, 58, 59
  proteasome capacity and demand, 58
  unfolded protein response, 61, 62
  X-BP1 expression, 58
Bruton tyrosine kinase (BTK) inhibitors, 25
  acalabrutinib, 17
  B cell development and lymphomagenesis, 3
  BCR signaling activation, 2
  BGB-3111, 18
  CC-292, 18
  CLL, 4, 5, 9
  combination treatments, 7
  CYP3A and CYP2D6, 5
  CYP3A4 inhibitors, 5
  development, 3
  ibrutinib, 4
  NEJM, 9
  ONO/GS4059, 17
  PK, 5
  role, 2
  structure, 3
  TEC kinase family, 3
  treatment, 3
  trials, CLL, 10–11
Burkitt lymphoma (BL), 115

C
Carfilzomib drug, 48
CD20+ lymphoproliferative disorders, 29
Cell extrinsic mechanisms

Cell extrinsic mechanisms (*cont.*)
 autophagy, 53, 54
 BCL-2 inhibitor, 56
 BMMSCs, 56
 efflux pumps, 52, 53
 hedgehog pathway, 57, 58
 interleukin-6, 57
 plasmacytic differentiation, 54, 55
 tumor microenvironment, 56
 proteasome subunit expression, 52, 55
Cerdulatinib, 123
Chronic lymphocytic leukemia (CLL)
 BCL2 inhibitors, 27, 35
 MCL, 38
 navitoclax testing, 34
 NHL, 25, 32
 patients, 33
 phase Ib study, 34
 rituximab, 38
 SLL, 28, 32, 35
 venetoclax killed CLL cells, 31, 37, 38
Circulating tumor DNA (ctDNA), 79
Common terminology criteria for adverse events (CTCAE), 77
Computational evolutionary models, 12
Cutaneous T-cell lymphoma (CTCL), 112
Cytokine-free environment, 108

D
Decitabine, 34
Diffuse large B cell lymphoma (DLBCL), 27, 47, 53, 54
 clinical indications and data, 77, 78
 mAbs, 74
 patients, 78
 R-CHOP regimen, 77
Dopamine receptor D-2 (DRD2), 62
Dose reductions, 5

E
EGFR/JAK/STAT3 pathway, 56
Epidermal growth factor receptor (EGFR), 55
Eukaryotic translation initiation factor 2 α (EIF2α), 50
Everolimus (RAD001), 85, 96, 97

F
Fedratinib, 123
Freedom from progression (FFP), 33

G
G1097 substitutions, 113
Genetic tumor heterogeneity, 93
Germinal center B-cell-like type (GCB) DLBCL, 77
 vs. non-GCB, 78
Gray zone lymphoma (GZL), 112
GRP78 oligomerization, 61

H
Hans classification, 77
Heat-shock protein 90 (HSP90), 125
Hedgehog pathway (Hh), 57, 58
Histone deacetylase 6 (HDAC6), 54
Hodgkin lymphoma (HL), 25, 28
Hyperglicemia, 91
Hyperlipidemia, 91

I
Ibrutinib, 4–8, 25, 32, 33, 35, 37
Idelalisib, 25
IMBRUVICA®, 4
Immunoglobulin variable heavy chain (IGVH) gene, 25
Immunomodulatory drugs (IMiDs)
 malignancies, 80
 MET/MEK inhibition, 80
 molecular mechanisms, 79, 80
 preclinical and clinical models, 80
 R2ICE, 80
Immunoproteasome, 48, 55, 56
Integrated stress response (ISR), 61
Interferon-gamma (INF-γ), 76
Interferon regulatory factor 4 (IRF4), 54
Interleukin-6 (IL-6), 57
IκB kinase (IKK), 48–50

J
JAK2I682F mutation, 126
JAK inhibitors, 120, 125
JAK2 mutations, 126
JAK2 pharmacological inhibition, 112
JAK/STAT pathway, 109, 119, 125
 chemical structure, 121
 FERM domain mutations, 113
 gene mutations, 111
 HL cells, 115
 IRAK1 and IRAK4 kinases, 116
 JAK2V617F mutation, 113
 JH1 and JH2 domains, 108

Index 137

JMJDC2, 112
lymphomagenesis signaling, 110–118
mediated signaling, 118
MYD88 mutations, 116
PMBCL and HL, 110
proteins, 110
PTPN11 activity, 116
PTPN1/PTPN2 mutations, 115
signaling pathway, 107–110
SOCS proteins, 108
STAT proteins, 114
Janus associated kinase (JAK), 55

K
78-kDa glucose regulated protein (GRP78), 50

L
Lenalidomide, 59
  IMiD pomalidomide, 79
  and lymphoma, 74, 75
  mAb Rituximab, 78
  myelodysplastic syndrome, 80
  NHL, 78
  preclinical models, 77
  predictive markers, 78
  structure and mechanism, 75, 76
  toxicities, 76, 77
Lestaurtinib, 124
Low molecular weight heparin (LMWH), 76
Lymphoma
  associated JAK1 mutations, 112, 116
  direct effects, 76
  DLBCL, 77
  follicular, 80
  liquid biopsies, 80
  myeloma cell lines, 77
  patients, 77
  treatment, 74, 75

M
Mammalian target of rapamycin (mTOR) inhibitors
  compounds, 85
  lipids and glucose, 91
  in lymphomas, 94
  mIAS, 92
  mutations, 92–93
  NSAIDs, 92
  PI3K/AKT pathway, 86
  rapamycin and rapalogs, 89
  second generation, 87, 88, 98–99

signaling pathways, 86
temsirolimus, 85
Mantle cell lymphoma (MCL), 27, 47, 51, 54, 55, 57–59, 61, 62, 86, 115
  efficacy and safety data, 7
  functional analysis, 9
  parameters, 9
  resistance mechanisms, 8–9, 15, 16
Marginal zone lymphoma (MZL), 8, 34
Minimal residual disease (MRD), 7, 33
Momelitinib drug, 124
mTOR innibitors associated stomatitis (mIAS), 92
mTOR resistance mutations, 88
Mucosa-associated lymphoid tissue (MALT) lymphoma, 116
Myelodysplastic syndrome, 79, 80
Myeloid differentiation primary response 88 (MYD88), 78
Myeloproliferative neoplasms (MPNs), 113

N
Navitoclax
  ABT-263, 28
  BCL2 selective inhibitor, 30
  BCLxL, 30
  bendamustine and rituximab, 29
  CD20+ lymphoproliferative disorders, 29
  clinical and preclinical data, 30
  clinical development, 30
  CLL/SLL, 28
  phase I trial, 30
  plus rituximab, 29
  relapsed/refractory B cell malignancies, 28
Nelfinavir, 61
Neutropenia, 76
New England Journal of Medicine (NEJM), 9
New-onset diabetes mellitus (NODM), 91
Nodal marginal zone lymphoma (NMZL), 118
Non-germinal B-cell-like type (non-GCB)
  vs. GCB, 78
  patients, 78
  subtype, 77
Non-Hodgkin's lymphoma (NHL), 47, 74
Nuclear factor kappa B (NFκB), 48, 50

O
Ohio State trial, 6
Oligomerization, 50
ONO/GS4059 (BTK inhibitor), 17

P

Pacritinib, 122
Peptidyl arginine deaminase (PADI), 57
Pharmacokinetic (PK) parameters, 5
Phosphatidylserine exposure, 30
Phosphoinositide 3 kinase (PI3κ) inhibitor, 25, 38
Plasmacytic differentiation, 54, 55
Pneumonitis, 90
Pomalidomide, 54
Primary mediastinal B-cell lymphoma (PMBCL), 110
Pro-apoptotic BH3-only proteins, 26
Progression free survival (PFS), 28, 33, 35, 37, 38
Pro-survival BCL2 proteins, 27
Proteasome inhibitors, 52–62
    anti-tumor effect, 48–51
    bortezomib resistance (see Bortezomib resistance)
    cell extrinsic mechanisms (see Cell extrinsic mechanisms)
    cell intrinsic mechanisms (see Cell intrinsic mechanisms)
    clinical trials, 63
    FDA approval, 47
    TJP1, 62
    ubiquitin, 47, 48
Pseudokinase, 108
Pump P-glycoprotein (PGP), 52, 53

R

Rapalogs, 89–90
Rapamycin, 85, 89
Redistribution lymphocytosis, 4
Regulatory-associated protein of mTOR (RAPTOR), 87
RESONATE trial, 6, 12
RESONATE-2 trial, 6
Retinoids, 60
Retrospective analysis, 15
Revlimid drug, 75
Richter' syndrome, 7, 9, 17
Ridaforolimus (MK-8669), 85, 87, 98
Rituximab, ifosfamide, carboplatin and etoposide (R-ICE), 78
Ruxolitinib, 120–122

S

SH2B3 frame-shift mutations, 116
Signalosome, 2
Signal-transducer-and-activator-of-transcription (STAT), 108
Signal transducer and activator of transcription 3 (STAT3), 55
Small lymphocytic lymphoma (SLL), 28
Somatic JAK2 mutations, 113
Sonic hedgehog (SHH), 57
Sonidegib, 60
STAT activation, 119
STAT3 anti-sense oligonucleotide inhibitors, 119–120
STAT5B mutations, 114
STAT3 phosphorylation, 114
STAT6 mutations, 114
β5 Subunit of the proteasome (PSMB5), 52
Suppressors-of-cytokine-signaling (SOCS) family, 108

T

T-cell lymphoblastic lymphoma (T-LBL), 113
Temsirolimus (CCI-779), 85, 87, 95, 96
Thalidomide, 54
Thrombocytopenia, 76, 92
Thromboprophylaxis, 77
Tight junction protein 1 (TJP1), 55
Tofacitinib, 120, 123
Topical ruxolitinib treatment, 121
Tumor lysis syndrome (TLS), 32
Tumor necrosis factor alpha (TNF-α), 76
Type-II JAK inhibitors, 125–127

U

Ubiquitin proteasome system, 47, 53
Unfolded protein response (UPR), 50, 58, 61, 62

V

Venetoclax
    administration and pharmacokinetics, 32
    biochemistry, 30
    clinical outcomes, 32–34
    pre-clinical data, 31, 32
    resistance
        clinical effect, 35
        molecular mechanisms, 35–38
Vismodegib, 60

W

Waldenstrom's macroglobulinemia (WM), 16, 27, 47, 97
Whole exome sequencing (WES), 9

X

X-box binding protein 1 (XBP-1), 50

Printed by Printforce, the Netherlands